THE IMPACT OF MANAGED CARE ON THE PRACTICE OF PSYCHOTHERAPY

Innovation, Implementation, and Controversy

THE IMPACT OF MANAGED CARE ON THE PRACTICE OF PSYCHOTHERAPY

Innovation, Implementation, and Controversy

Edited by

Richard M. Alperin, D.S.W., B.C.D

and

David G. Phillips, D.S.W., B.C.D

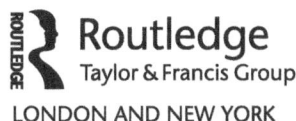

Routledge
Taylor & Francis Group

LONDON AND NEW YORK

First published 1997 by Brunner/Mazel, Inc.

Published 2018 by Routledge
2 Park Square, Milton Park, Abingdon, Oxon OX14 4RN
52 Vanderbilt Avenue, New York, NY 10017

First issued in paperback 2018

Routledge is an imprint of the Taylor & Francis Group, an informa business

Library of Congress Cataloging-in-Publication Data
The impact of managed care on the practice of psychotherapy:
  innovation, implementation, and controversy / edited by Richard M.
  Alperin and David G. Phillips
      p.   cm.
  Includes bibliographical references and index.
  ISBN 0-87630-830-2
  1. Managed mental health care.   I. Alperin, Richard M.
II. Phillips, David G., D.S.W.
RC465.5.I47   1997
616.89′14–dc20   96-41932
                                                      CIP

ISBN-13: 978-1-138-87176-2 (pbk)
ISBN-13: 978-0-87630-830-1 (hbk)

Contents

The Editors

Richard M. Alperin, D.S.W., B.C.D. Full-time private practice in Teaneck, New Jersey and New York City; Adjunct Associate Professor, Fordham University Graduate School of Social Service; Faculty: Object Relations Institute for Psychotherapy and Psychoanalysis; Psychoanalytic Psychotherapy Study Center; New Jersey Institute for Training in Psychoanalysis. Former Chair, Committee on Psychoanalysis, New York State Society for Clinical Social Work.

David G. Phillips, D.S.W., B.C.D. Training and Supervising Analyst, Psychoanalytic Institute of the Postgraduate Center for Mental Health; Adjunct Associate Professor, Wurzweiler School of Social Work, Yeshiva University; Co-Chair, Committee on Professional Standards, National Federation of Societies for Clinical Social Work; President-Elect, National Membership Committee on Psychoanalysis in Clinical Social Work; Distinguished Practitioner in Social Work, National Academies of Practice; Private practice in New York City and New Jersey.

Contributing Authors

Helen Altman, M.S.W., B.C.D. Marriage and family therapist, with post-graduate certificates from The Ackerman Institute in Family Therapy and Smith College School for Social Work. Served on numerous state committees and task forces, including member of the Board of Visitors for Harlem Valley Psychiatric Center. Published author and presenter at numerous national conferences on diverse subjects including Family Therapy with Hospitalized Patients; Collaborative Discharge Planning, a research model for the chronically mentally ill. Private practice in White Plains, New York.

William Ballen, C.S.W. Director of Clinical Services, The Institute for Hypnosis Research and Psychotherapy of the Morton Prince Centers for Hypnotherapy; Instructor, The Society for Clinical and Experimental Hypnosis; chair, Clinical Hypnosis Practice Committee, New York State Society for Clinical Social Work; Board Certified in Pain Management, The American Academy of Pain Management; Diplomate in Behavioral Medicine, International Society of Behavioral Medicine; Ph.D. Candidate (A.B.D.) in Psychology, California Coast University; Full-time private practice, Long Beach, New York.

Susan Birne-Stone, M.S.W. Account Executive, Merit Behavioral Care Corp.; Ph.D. candidate, New York University School of Social Work; private practice in New York City.

Adrienne Cypres, M.A., M.S.W., Ph.D. School of Social Work; private practice in New York City.

Joyce Edward, M.S.W., B.C.D. Contributing editor, Clinical Social Work Journal; coauthor; *Separation-Individuation Theory and Application;* Co-founder and past Co-Chair, Coalition of Mental Health Professionals and Consumers; Distinguished Practitioner in Social Work, National Academies of Practice; private practice of psychotherapy and psychoanalysis; Coeditor, *Fostering Healing and Growth: A Psychoanalytic Social Work Approach* (1996), New York: Jason Aronson.

Kenneth A. Frank, Ph.D. Co-Founder and Director of Training, National Institute for the Psychotherapies; Clinical Professor in Psychiatry, Columbia University College of Physicians and Surgeons; author and lecturer on analytic therapy; private practice in New York City and Englewood, New Jersey.

Sidney Grossberg, M.S.W., Ph.D., B.C.D. Executive Director, Counseling Associates, Southfield, Michigan; faculty, Continuing Education and Postgraduate Certificate programs, Smith College School for Social Work; national consultant on managed care and forming and expanding behavioral group practices; advisory boards of managed care and insurance companies; Distinguished Practitioner in Social Work, National Academies of Practice.

William G. Herron, Ph.D. Professor, Department of Psychology, St. John's University; Senior Supervisor and Training Analyst, Contemporary Center for Advanced Psychoanalytic Studies; coauthor, *Narcissism and the Psychotherapist* and *Money Matters: The Fee in Psychotherapy and Psycho-analysis;* private practice.

Kent Jarratt, A.C.S.W. Director of Hypnotherapy Services, the National Institute for the Psychotherapies. He is a former Board Member of the New York Milton H. Erickson Society for Psychotherapy and Hypnosis. He is affiliated with the Center for the Study of Anorexia and Bulimia and is a staff consultant for the Lesbian and Gay Community Services Center in Manhattan, where he also maintains a private practice.

Kelley Phillips, M.D., M.P.H. President, Institute for Research on Women's Health, Washington, D.C.; former Medical Director for the Office of Quality Assurance, American Psychiatric Association, Washington, D.C.

Steven A. Rosenberg, Ph.D. Assistant Professor, Department of Psychiatry, University of Colorado Health Sciences Center; former Senior Psychologist, Kaiser Permanente Mental Health Sevices, Charlotte, N.C.

Steven Winderbaum, M.S.W. Clinician, Merit Behavioral Care Corp.;

former social service trainer and faculty, Cornell University, and City University of New York; Adjunct Associate Professor, Touro College, School of General Studies; private practice in New York City.

Phyllis Wright, M.S.W., B.C.D. President, Eastern Group Psychotherapy Society; Dean of Admissions, Group Therapy Training Program of Eastern Group Psychotherapy Society; Supervisor and Teacher of Group Therapy, Postgraduate Center for Mental Health, Training Institute for Mental Health Practitioners, Eastern Group Psychotherapy Association; private practice in New York City.

Introduction

As managed care networks increasingly dominate the provision of health care in the United States, all practitioners are being affected by the principles and practices of these organizations. Some professionals in the mental health field, including those who work with alcohol- and drug-related disorders, have responded by leaving practice altogether, or by reorganizing and refocusing their work so that they will not have to function within the requirements and constraints of managed care systems. Other practitioners have welcomed the advent of managed care, hoping, perhaps, that referrals from managed care companies will enhance their private practices, and they have attempted to join as many managed care networks as possible. Whether the development of managed care is greeted with pleasure, indifference, or hostility, there is general agreement that the practice of psychotherapy will be irrevocably changed, since managed care has drastically altered the delivery, definition, and outcome of the psychotherapy that patients receive under its aegis (Bozutto, 1992).

Currently there are over two hundred managed care companies serving approximately half the population of the United States; it is anticipated that within the next two or three years this figure will approach the entire population covered by insurance benefits (Bozutto, 1992). As a result, even those psychotherapists who deplore managed care have found it necessary to become involved with some of these systems so as not to deprive their patients of needed insurance coverage or to assure the survival and continuity of their private practices. For most psychotherapists, however, this adjustment has not been easy. While certain practitioners, such as those practicing short-term therapy, have found it relatively simple to integrate managed care requirements into their existing practices, others, such as psychoanalytically oriented therapists, are outraged and feel that their professional autonomy has been curtailed, since the limitations of managed care prevent them from offering the type of treatment they believe to be both necessary and responsible. In order to advance an understanding of the practice of psychotherapy in the era of managed care and to aid practitioners in functioning effectively within these systems, this volume presents practitioners representing a variety of viewpoints discussing their experiences, concerns, and predictions about managed care.

THE DEVELOPMENT OF MANAGED CARE

Psychotherapists who are troubled by the advent of managed care may be surprised to learn that it had its origin in the "democratic intent to bring health care to populations of people at an affordable cost" (Bennett, 1988, p. 1544). This was the early emphasis of the health maintenance organization (HMO) movement, the evolution of which may be traced to two different sources. The first of these, prepayment, or the provision of a set package of health care services by an identifiable provider for a preestablished fee, originated in the Pacific Northwest in the early 1900s. Industrial workers in remote areas lacked adequate medical care, and their employers provided for this care by utilizing salaried physicians. Group practice, the other source of the development of HMOs, was introduced in the 1880s by the Mayo brothers, who sought to improve the quality of patient care by bringing together a variety of specialists capable of approaching a patient's problems from a plurality of perspectives and of coordinating care within one organizational setting (Bittker, 1992). It was not until 1929, however, that the final element of the modern HMO, prepayment for services, was combined with the organizational development of group practices.

With the Great Society programs of the 1960s, and the development of Medicare and Medicaid in 1965, the government began to pay directly for the provision of health services, and there was growing concern that all citizens have proper health care. Increased governmental involvement and the effort to provide health services to larger segments of the population were important factors as the costs of health care began to grow rapidly out of control. This rise in costs served as the inspiration for the formation of alternative health care delivery systems (Bennett, 1988).

The Kaiser Permanente Health Plan, organized in the 1930s, served as the model for many of the health care experiments of the 1960s which later developed into staff and group HMOs. Encouraged by their focus on the prevention as well as the treatment of illness, and their provision of affordable and accessible health care to large populations, the federal government endorsed the development of HMOs by passing the Health Maintenance Act of 1973. This act led to the proliferation of HMOs by offering them low-cost loans and grants and by decreasing certain legal restrictions that were inhibiting further expansion (Austad & Berman, 1991). The increased availability of funds and the relaxation of legal controls combined to encourage profit-making corporations to enter the health maintenance field (Dowart & Epstein, 1992).

While HMOs were initially maverick forms of health care delivery with a populist flavor (Harron & Adlerstein, 1994) that often operated on a non-profit basis, most are now large, complex, profit-making corporations operating within a highly competitive health care market (Winegar & Bistline, 1994). As Starr (1982) has stated, "The socialized medicine of one era has become the corporate reform of the next" (p. 396).

While several basic HMO models have been introduced over the years, currently they tend to fall into three general categories. The first, known as the staff model, offers its subscribers comprehensive medical services by salaried providers within the confines of a health center. The second, the group model, constitutes a number of practitioners incorporated into a group who have a contract with the HMO to provide its subscribers with specific services, usually from a centralized location (Vizza, 1987). In the third, referred to as the independent practice model, the health care professionals have a contract with the HMO to provide services to its subscribers from their own private offices. Providers are reimbursed in these last two models by the HMO on a prearranged fee-for-service basis or through a capitation payment per patient, regardless of the frequency of visits or the services provided (Austad & Berman, 1991).

To further contain the costs of health care in this country, preferred provider organizations (PPOs) have also been introduced (Gurevitz, 1986). These organizations can best be described as intermediaries between the health care consumer and the insurance company or employer sponsoring the insurance. In a PPO, the consumer is able to select the health care professional from a panel, which provides services to subscribers at a discounted fee. Through these reduced fees and careful review of how services are utilized, there is an effort to reduce the costs of health care (Vizza, 1987).

When experimentation with new forms of health care delivery began in 1965, there was already great concern about the costs of health care, even though expenditures on health care were less than 6% of our gross national domestic spending. Since that time this cost has escalated rapidly; in the early 1990s, it exceeded 12%. Considering that by the beginning of the twenty-first century the cost of health care is expected to exceed 15% of our gross national spending (Gray, 1991), all parties agree that this cost is out of control. Organizations such as HMOs and PPOs have become increasingly popular as part of the efforts to contain these costs, and they have been subsumed under the general category of "managed care" as one important part of the effort to solve the health care crisis in this country.

MENTAL HEALTH SERVICES AND MANAGED CARE

Most of the early HMOs did not include benefits for the treatment of mental illness; therefore managed mental health care is relatively new. After a number of pilot studies in the early 1960s demonstrated that limited mental health benefits were affordable, HMOs were pressured by large contractor groups to include such treatment on an optional basis. As provision of this benefit proved to be feasible, new HMO plans in the late 1960s began to include mental health care as a basic benefit (Bennett, 1988).

In order to qualify for federal assistance, the Health Maintenance Act of 1973 required plans to provide up to 20 outpatient sessions per year for evaluation and crisis intervention. Although this law did not require benefits for inpatient psychiatric care, most new HMO plans included benefits for 30 to 45 days of inpatient care or partial care for 60 to 90 days (Bittker, 1992).

Most insurance companies have been hesitant to include mental health benefits in their plans out of concern about the costs of such treatment. Mental health care comprises as much as 25% of all health care costs, and is the third largest source of health-related expenses (Austad & Berman, 1991). It should be noted, however, that the great majority of these costs are for services to the chronically mentally ill and for inpatient care rather than for outpatient psychotherapy.

In spite of these costs, at least 40 states have now required insurance companies to provide benefits covering mental health treatment. Although these benefits differ by state and include multiple levels of coverage limitations, these laws emphasize, in general, inpatient rather than outpatient mental health benefits (Levin & Glasser, 1992).

Most insurance companies have been reluctant to offer outpatient psychotherapy benefits, fearing that this would create a "moral hazard." That is, they were concerned that inclusion of such benefits would lead subscribers to be more likely to utilize these services, and that this would result in exorbitant costs that they could not afford (Dorwart & Epstein, 1992).

What has been discovered through extensive research, however, is that outpatient psychotherapy is cost-effective, since it reduces the use of general medical services and the consequent expenditures for such treatment (Austad & Berman, 1991). In addition, outpatient psychotherapy can frequently prevent hospitalization for mental illness, which is much more expensive and, as noted, is one the major factors responsible for the high cost of mental health care in this country. Furthermore, as they became aware of the detrimental impact that psychological problems and substance abuse have upon productivity, employers discovered that outpatient psychotherapy was cost-effective for them and that psychotherapy was an effective form of treatment for such problems (Winegar & Bistline, 1994).

As employees and the general public began increasingly to request that mental health benefits be included in their coverage, insurance companies began to realize that in order to market their policies successfully, they would have to offer such benefits. But they were still faced with the problem of how to offer such benefits without incurring a "moral hazard." Strategies that have attempted to prevent such overutilization have included large deductibles and copayments (payments that must be made by subscribers in order to utilize their insurance benefits); delays in treatment; limits on the care that is covered; and the current approach of managed care, which includes utilization management and limiting the duration and frequency of psychotherapy (Dorwart & Epstein, 1992).

WHAT IS MANAGED MENTAL HEALTH CARE?

In spite of the growth of managed care in recent years, there is no consensual agreement within the industry or among health care providers as to the exact definition of managed care. Goodman and colleagues (1992) broadly define it as patient care that is determined by external review procedures rather than exclusively by the practitioner. These external review procedures are referred to as "utilization management," which has been defined as a "set of techniques used by or on behalf of the purchaser of health benefits to manage health care costs by influencing patient care decision making through a case by case assessment of care prior to its provision" (Institute of Medicine, 1989, p. 17).

Winegar and Bistline (1994) have provided an excellent definition of managed care within the field of mental health as "the systems and technologies aimed at organizing and managing both the clinical and financial services to a given population of consumers" (p. 17). Managed care firms were established to perform these functions, but originally they served only HMOs and insurance companies. In the late 1980s, several large, self-insured companies, such as IBM, which were concerned about the mental health needs of their employees, began to contract directly with managed mental health care companies. Managed care firms even established and provided employee assistance programs for some of these employer companies (Winegar, 1992). Of the more than two hundred current managed care companies, many are national in scope, and they are usually owned by large insurance companies (Bozzuto, 1992). Although this industry is only 15 years old, it has already produced an annual revenue in excess of a billion dollars (Winegar & Bistline, 1994).

These managed care companies have established and maintained large networks of mental health professionals and facilities who have agreed, through a formal contract, to provide eligible patients with services at a discounted fee and to comply with the companies' utilization management procedures (Winegar & Bistline, 1994). Most of these mental health professionals are community providers and have received an orientation to the managed care company's philosophy of treatment.

A variety of utilization management procedures are administered by these companies. They include preadmission screening and/or precertification of treatment; close monitoring of ongoing treatment and regular review of its progress; and, when appropriate, discharge planning. While these procedures are both complex and expensive to administer, they are designed to both reduce the costs of mental health care and improve the quality of the treatment.

PSYCHOTHERAPY IN MANAGED CARE

Most current mental health professionals were trained prior to the development of managed care; often, they do not feel intellectually or emotionally prepared to work within the new environment. In addition, many practitioners, such as psychoanalysts and psychoanalytic psychotherapists, practice modalities of treatment they feel do not fit into a managed care context. At the same time, however, numerous practitioners have become providers for numerous managed care networks, both out of economic necessity and to make sure that their patients receive the insurance benefits to which they are entitled.

The fact that each managed care company has its own administrative procedures and treatment guidelines adds to the frustration and bewilderment that practitioners often feel. Even within the same company, the instructions for their work may vary, since these guidelines are partially based upon the various contracts that the managed care company has with the particular patient's employer or insurance carrier (Neuwirth, 1993).

Despite specific differences, however, all managed care companies seem to share a general preference for a philosophy of treatment and style of practice. They conceive of the managed care psychotherapist as a "psychological family doctor" (Austad & Berman, 1991), similar to the family physician who becomes familiar with the patient and/or family and provides treatment for brief episodes over an extended period of time (Patterson & Berman, 1991).

Since this managed care model requires the most "efficient, effective, parsimonious and minimally intrusive therapeutic interventions" (Austad & Berman, 1991, p. 12), delivered intermittently, when necessary, throughout the life of the patient, various short-term strategies, such as the "solution focused" approach are recommended (Winegar, 1992). There has, therefore, been a convergence in most managed care plans in allowing for 20 outpatient psychotherapy sessions per person per year, as long as they are found to be medically necessary (Levin & Glasser, 1992).

Irrespective of the limit of the psychotherapy benefit, all managed care organizations require careful monitoring and review of this treatment. Some companies are more restrictive in the procedures they employ, such as screening all potential patients before they start treatment and/or requiring frequent utilization reviews after every few sessions. Other companies are more liberal, requiring utilization review only after a significant time period, such as every few months.

Many psychotherapists object to these procedures, arguing that they intrude into the confidential relationship between therapist and patient, and adversely affect the outcome of the treatment (Gabbard et al., 1991). Others have objected to the brevity of the treatment, arguing that it is "mere" crisis intervention, that short-term treatment is not appropriate for everyone, and that such treatment is, at best, a superficial remedy (Bozutto, 1992; Shore, 1992). Other psychotherapists have criticized managed care for abandoning its original goal of bringing affordable health care to the underserved and focusing, instead, on its own profits (Bennett, 1988).

This volume offers contributions to the debate over managed care from the experience of psychotherapists on both sides of the controversy. It is evident from these papers that some psychotherapists are fitting comfortably into a managed care environment and are finding the opportunity to extend the type of treatment that they have always practiced. It is also evident that others are finding it difficult to function within this environment, which demands new skills, a new type of practice, and a revision of their beliefs about what constitutes appropriate treatment. The advent of managed care is affecting every aspect of the practice of psychotherapy, and all practitioners want to continue to provide the highest quality of service within its framework. It is hoped that this volume will contribute to all psychotherapists' understanding of the world of managed care practice and that it will help them to meet its challenges.

Richard M. Alperin
David G. Phillips

REFERENCES

Austad, C. S., & Berman, W. H. (1991). Managed health care and the evolution of psychotherapy. In C. S. Austad & W. H. Berman (Eds.), *Psychotherapy in managed health care: The optimal use of time and resources.* Washington, DC: American Psychological Association, pp. 3–19.

Bennett, M. J. (1988). The greening of the HMO: Implications for prepaid psychiatry. *American Journal of Psychiatry, 145,* 1544–1549.

Bittker, T. E. (1992). The emergence of prepaid psychiatry. In J. L. Feldman & R. J. Fitzpatrick (Eds.), *Managed mental health care: Administrative and clinical issues* (pp. 3–10). Washington, DC: American Psychiatric Press.

Bozzuto, J. (1992). Psychoanalysis in the world of managed care. Presented at the American Academy of Psychoanalysis, December 1992.

Dorwart, R. A., & Epstein, S. S. (1992). Economics and managed mental health care: The HMO as a crucible for cost-effective care. In J. L. Feldman & R. J. Fitzpatrick (Eds.), *Managed mental health care: Administrative and clinical issues* (pp. 11–27). Washington, DC: American Psychiatric Press.

Gabbard, G., Tetsuro T., Davison, J., Bauman-Bork, M., & Ensroth, K. (1991). A psychodynamic perspective on the clinical impact of insurance review. *American Journal of Psychiatry, 148,* 318–323.

Goodman, M., Brown, J., & Dietz, P. (1992). *Managing managed care: A mental health practitioner's survivor guide.* Washington, DC: American Psychiatric Press.

Gray, B. (1991). *The profit motive and patient care.* Cambridge, MA: Harvard University Press.

Gurevitz, H. (1986). Preferred provider organizations and psychiatric treatment. In D. W. Krueger (Ed.), *The last taboo: Money as symbol and reality in psychotherapy and psychoanalysis.* New York: Brunner/Mazel, pp. 244–252.

Harron, W. G., & Alderstein, L. K. (1994). The dynamics of managed mental health care. *Psychological Reports, 75,* 723–741.

Institute of Medicine (U.S.). (1989). *Committee on utilization management by third parties: Controlling costs and changing patient care: The role of utilization management.* M. J. Field & Gray, B. H. (Eds.). Washington, D.C.: National Academy Press.

Levin, B. L., & Glasser, J. H. (1992). Comparing mental health benefits, utilization patterns, and costs. In J. L. Feldman & R. J. Fitzpatrick (Eds.), *Managed mental health care: Administrative and clinical issues.* Washington, DC: American Psychiatric Press, pp. 29–52.

Neuwirth, E. (1993). What does managed care want from us? A psychotherapist's guide to survival. Keynote address presented at the 25th anniversary conference of the New York State Society for Clinical Social Work.

Patterson, D., & Berman, W. (1991). Organizational and service delivery issues in managed mental health services. In C. S. Austad & W. H. Berman (Eds.), *Psychotherapy in managed health care: The optimal use of time and resources* (pp. 19–32). Washington, DC: American Psychological Association.

Shore, K. (1992). Managed care: What you can do? *Adelphi Society of Psychoanalysis and Psychotherapy Newsletter, 6,* 6–7.

Starr, P. (1982). *The social transformation of American medicine.* New York: Basic Books, p. 396.

Vizza, J. (1987). Psychologist participation in HMOs and PPOs. *Psychotherapy in Private Practice, 5,* 9–19.

Winegar, N. (1992). *The clinician's guide to managed mental health care.* New York: Haworth Press.

Winegar, N., & Bistline, J. (1994). *Marketing mental health services to managed care.* New York: Haworth Press.

PART I

Managed Care and Innovations in Psychotherapy Practice

As suggested in the introduction to this volume, managed care has created a revolution in the manner in which mental health and substance abuse services are organized and delivered. Many mental health professionals are not only deeply involved in this type of service delivery but are at the cutting edge of the current innovations; their experiences and views are presented in this section.

The development of managed care is concurrent with and fueled by another revolution—that of rapid and far-reaching transformations in the way that information is stored, processed, and transmitted. Kelley Phillips links these two revolutions in presenting a view of the future affected by these innovations. Her view, from inside the world of managed care, presents a compelling picture of what psychotherapists will need to know and do in order to both function in the current environment and prepare themselves for that which is just around the corner.

11

Another of the long-range effects of the managed care revolution is the increasing trend toward the development of multidisciplinary group practices. These groups, often preferred by managed care organizations, can provide a wider range of services than solo practitioners, can offer more systematic evaluations of the outcome of their work, and are better prepared to enter into the kinds of contractual and financial arrangements offered by managed care. Sidney Grossberg, a psychotherapist who has unusually extensive experience in this type of practice, offers specific suggestions for practitioners who may be interested in this type of option.

Every practitioner who has worked with managed care knows of the need to work with a case manager who represents the policies and interests of the company in monitoring work with the patient. Susan Birne-Stone, Adrienne Cypres, and Steven Winderbaum are three experienced case managers who explore this relationship from a vantage point inside the managed care organization. They discuss such key issues as the meaning and importance of utilization review and medical necessity and the role of the case manager in assessment and treatment.

Another important and often controversial effect of the managed care revolution has been the increasing stress on the use of psychoactive drugs in treatment. Managed care companies often feel that these drugs have clearly proven their usefulness in a scientifically acceptable manner and that they are more cost-effective than prolonged psychotherapy. In her second chapter, Kelley Phillips provides a specific outline for psychotherapists to consider in determining whether or not a psychiatric evaluation is appropriate.

R.M.A.
D.G.P.

CHAPTER 1

Preparing Ourselves as Behavioral Health Clinicians for the Twenty-First Century

Kelley L. Phillips

For many practitioners, particularly in the *behavioral health* field, these are anxious times as we close out this century. The very foundation of our training, core knowledge, skills, and livelihood are being tremendously challenged. It seems that our time-honored clinical teaching, training, and supervision have not kept pace to assist us with and inform us of the very different demands of delivering behavioral health care today. We have a new lexicon, terms such as *managed care, provider groups, outcomes, networks*. We require new evaluative, *quantitative*, and *qualitative* skills as well as new tools such as laptop computers to give us online information that will enable us to deliver our care as efficiently and effectively as possible.

The healing arts are being transformed so that scientific rigor is more in evidence in clinical practice. The best treatments are still in demand, but *best* is being redefined. This term once referred to the most renowned, expensive, or chic clinician identified by patients and colleagues and promoted by word of mouth. Now *best* is determined more scientifically, using quantitative and qualitative measures, such as clinical decision analysis

---

Note: See the Appendix at the end of Chapter 4 (p. 73) for definitions of words that appear in *italics*.

(Detsky et al., 1994). This process includes evaluating optimal patient outcomes in the context of the most efficient use of resources. Thus, this "best treatment" can be compared reliably with other treatments to demonstrate its superiority. In addition, clinicians are being asked to demonstrate these findings to their patients to educate them about their role in maintaining their health. In parallel with these changes, clinicians are being reimbursed using this methodology by the public or a *third-party* payor. *Third party* is a medical insurance term used to designate the major payor of health services, which also determines the health benefits of the plan. Today, this payor is more likely to be a family member's employer or the federal government, which pays for Medicare, or the federal/state governments, which pay for Medicaid, rather than an insurance entity, which may contract with a third party and cut the checks for that party.

Another major trend in health care reform is the integration of behavioral health into the health care delivery system rather than maintaining a dual track. This direction is the result of the hard work done to decrease stigmatization of mental health care and *chemical dependence* and demonstrates that behavioral health has a significant impact on physical health. The converse is also true: physical disorders affect emotional well-being (Vandenbos & Deleon, 1988). For behavioral health clinicians, this trend underscores consideration of the entire person as well as integration of other health services when evaluation and treatment are offered. This approach is something new for many clinicians who provide psychotherapy independently of other treatments. They do not speak with psychiatrists (who provide psychotrophic medications for their patients) or consult with primary care physicians (who provide most of their patients' physical care). It is well demonstrated that coordinated care is better care, which utilizes resources more effectively (Hoeper, & Nyca, 1981; Borus et al. 1985). Coordinated care is also what we are being asked to provide and what will be paid for by a third party.

We are making great strides in the struggle to have behavioral health medicine receive parity of benefits with the rest of health care. Many health plans have a limited number of behavioral health benefits, such as 20 outpatient sessions per year, which does not occur in the medical-surgical component of the health plan. In return, we are being held to the same accountability standards as the rest of medicine; that is, we must demonstrate that our treatment interventions are effective and have a positive impact on the health status of our patients. These developments pose new challenges for those behavioral health clinicians who have not trained in the medical or public health sciences. The *biopsychosocial* model is defined as treating the whole person in the context of his or her family and community. This model is paired with a public health approach focusing on early intervention, education, and a coordinated health care delivery system. This framework incorporates a significant body of knowledge for clinicians to master.

If we consider these current health care trends from a "macro" perspective, we learn that these changes are expected and are bound to evolve given the history, sociology, and technology of American medicine and society (Starr, 1994, 1982). Four major trends are identified. First, the payors of health care want some clearer evidence that the services rendered, in the private relationship of patient–therapist, are effective and efficient. This response is due to the explosion of health care costs since the early eighties. Second is the dramatic increase in knowledge about the healing arts. New treatments are being developed at an incredible pace, with renewed attention to such complex areas as domestic violence and child abuse. Third is the global communications revolution, which provides instant information, shared with everyone, and thus creates a consumer demand that therapists provide state-of-the-art treatment. And fourth there is a demand for accountability that far surpasses the demand in previous times. These themes are integrated under the generic term *managed care*.

This chapter attempts to identify not only what we need in order to prepare ourselves but also how we might approach this essential transformation in health care if we want to survive as practicing clinicians. There are four fundamental principles/skills/tools that practitioners must learn and incorporate into their practices to succeed in the next decade and century. They are as follows:

- To effectively incorporate new information into our clinical practice in a timely manner
- To consider clinical resources as precious as one's own and therefore to develop a socially relevant cost/benefit analysis for every treatment intervention
- To use a public health approach to care that has as its principal foci early intervention and a coordinated continuum of health care services
- To evaluate the effectiveness of services delivered, thus facilitating positive change in a patient's health status

THE INFORMATION REVOLUTION: EFFECTIVE AND TIMELY

Our technological revolution in computers began in the early 1970s and, continues at a frenetic pace. The effect of this transformation is profoundly felt in health care. Gone are the days of scientific findings wending their way into clinical practice inconsistently over an interval of 10 or more years. It is imperative for clinicians to incorporate these findings into their practices in a timely and effective manner. It has been estimated that today a clinician becomes obsolete within an 18-month interval by not using information systems competently (Tyler, 1994).

Information technology is a new metaphor for our reality, with computers, software, and digital networks forming a magical bridge (Bunch & Hellemans, 1994). Our world is smaller and more manageable due to this global communications superhighway. In this realm, clinicians, specifically psychotherapists, have not kept pace with the rest of the world. The health care sector has been the slowest to adapt, with productivity increasing at a slow rate of 0.2% annually, compared with 4.6% for other work sectors (Bureau of Labor Statistics, 1991). Clinicians, especially psychotherapists, have been the last to adapt. This is partly a result of working in solo practices and not linking up to share information. Clinicians must catch up in this arena if they are to be successful in delivering clinical services effectively. Computer phobia is common among psychotherapists, who seem to have an antitechnical/antiscience bias. Basically, this stems from the conflict or division between the arts and science/technology. Many psychotherapists have traditionally focused more on the "art" of healing than on the science. It is clear that service delivery has to be both art and science to maximize an optimal outcome for our patients by the most efficient means possible (Kuhn, 1970).

Scientific information and its transfer are developing so fast that it is very difficult to keep up and manage it all. It is impossible without using information systems. Those clinicians who are newly graduated have grown up in this new age and are able to adapt readily. Those clinicians approaching retirement are frequently retiring early rather than grappling with this transition. However, it is the large middle group of clinicians who have been in practice 10 or more years who provide the majority of clinical services and who are experiencing the most distress in response to these changes. It is to this critical group that health care organizations, both managerial and service delivery systems, need to make their commitment.

The 1990s are identified as the "Decade of the Brain" (101st Congress, 1989), in which more clinical information has been discovered than in the previous two millennia. As science moves at breathtaking speed to provide new discoveries for our field, it is critical that clinicians be able to incorporate these breakthroughs into their practices as quickly and reliably as possible. There are many reasons to perform this rapid translation, but two important ones are (1) to provide state-of-the-art *effective* treatments for optimal patient outcomes, since only these treatments will be reimbursed, and (2) to utilize resources as *efficiently* as possible, since this is part of the outcome equation. The underlying assumptions are that as treatments are continuously refined and improved, clinicians need to be constantly in a learning mode. As well, clinicians have acquired a new responsibility in delivering health care: they must consider treatments from a *cost/benefit* perspective. This approach is very different than the traditional fee-for-service model, where the incentive axiom is "more is better"—more services, more technology, more clinicians, more out-of-control costs and consumption, but not necessarily better outcomes. In the fee-for-service model, the real costs of health care have been hidden from the consumer as well as from the clinician, since the majority of costs have been paid by third parties—federal and state governments as well as employer groups (Starr, 1994).

How can we incorporate this massive explosion of clinical information at a time when there are tremendous demands for us to provide increasingly refined clinical services faster and better? Similarly, we are expected not just to proffer but truly to evaluate our effectiveness and cost of treatment. We need to learn new skills to be able to meet these demands. No longer is there tolerance for clinical research that languishes in the lab and is not quickly integrated into clinical practice. Clinicians are expected to take the lead in this implementation. Scientists will also be expected to focus on the implications and implementation of their findings into the service delivery systems. These new expectations will of necessity create linkages between science and its applications. Our information and communication systems are the major tools to make this happen.

What will our practices look like if we succeed in dealing with the information explosion?

Personal computers will be on our desks and we will have comprehensive software packages that will include practice guidelines and parameters for different diagnoses, clinical issues, and problems as well as a help line for consultation on clinical issues. A display field will show us the progress of a particular patient in comparison with other patients with the same severity, comparative risk factors, and problems. On-line consultation will be available for managing polypharmacy, drug interactions, specific patient profiles, and physical illnesses. Demographic data will be available to identify clinicians, types of treatment, success rates, and costs for referral services.

Physically, more of our offices will be configured with those of other clinicians who provide complementary services. For example, a primary care group will include behavioral health clinicians who provide the spectrum of services—child and family, trauma sequelae, depression, psychopharmacology, and chemical dependence.

How will we be able to link up? Organized medicine such as health maintenance organizations (HMOs), preferred provider groups (PPOs), and provider networks have taken the lead in using information systems to incorporate practice parameters, clinician profiling, and costs of services. Information displayed is relatively easy to understand given the assumption that a clinician has mastered the basics of using a personal computer and understands health statistics such as the variance in practice patterns, the specific kinds of patient outcomes, and the reliability and validity of data. Courses in health statistics are available at schools of public health and in programs and schools training in health care. Personal computer generations are occurring at rates of at least yearly periodicity. Computer journals, magazines, your children, and friendly techies may assist you in making your selection.

COST/BENEFIT ANALYSIS

What do we mean by cost/benefit analysis? How do we evaluate it? Before a definition of *cost/benefit analysis* is given, it is useful to define the terms *efficiency* and *effectiveness* as used in health care. A treatment for a specific patient with a particular health problem or diagnosis is effective when the treatment brings about a positive change in the health status of the patient: the outcome for the patient is improved. The efficiency of this treatment is measured by considering the costs involved in delivering the services for this problem. *Optimal treatment* is defined as the most effective treatment delivered using the most efficient resources. Consider a patient with a diagnosis of major depression of moderate severity where suicide impulsivity is minimal. One treatment choice is interpersonal psychotherapy (ITP), medication, family assessment, and family education in an outpatient setting over a period of 3 months. The patient and family are much improved, as measured by the patient's improved mood, sleep pattern, involvement in family activities, and work performance; this is reflected in the rating scales that measure level of depression. Another treatment of the same problem, severity, and circumstances involves hospitalizing the patient for 25 days, making no family assessment and little effort to coordinate outpatient and inpatient treatments. If we consider a cost/benefit analysis of these two approaches at the end of the third month of treatment, we find that the direct costs of payment of services are 17 times higher for the inpatient approach (calculation based on a cost of $800 per hospital day—that is, 25 days times $800, versus 12 outpatient sessions at $100 per session); with greater risk of job loss due to patient absenteeism, increased family stress caused by dealing with a family member in the hospital, and more physician and allied professional resources utilized.

Clinicians are the main decision makers in determining what kind and how much health care will be delivered to patients. Clinicians are not only responsible for identifying treatment options but also for delivering those treatments. The first part of this decision tree is to determine the nature of the patient's problem and then to consider what treatment options there are, if any, and which one will be the most effective in the context of available resources. Consider, for example, a patient with a family problem who is treated with individual psychotherapy, the treatment that the clinician knows how to deliver best. This type of psychotherapy is not optimal treatment for this problem and the resources invested are mismatched. The result is that resources are used inefficiently in the short term, wasting time and money and adversely affecting the family's well-being; in the long term, family distress is prolonged, which affects job stress, performance, and security. It is estimated that we are still wasting about one-third of our health care dollars by delivering care inefficiently (Gray & Field, 1989). This depletes funds that would be available to provide excellent care for all citizens, including about 40 million Americans presently not covered (Health Insurance Association of America, 1994).

Another example of problematic practice is how most physicians, including psychiatrists, learn about new drugs. Most obtain their information from pharmaceutical company representatives. There are several problems with this commercial method. First, much of the "research" distributed by drug companies to demonstrate the superior effects of a particular drug is of poor quality. The methodology is poor, with either no control groups and just another drug group compared, no double-blind design to maximize objectivity of findings, no replication of the study using a large enough sample, drug duration and follow-up too brief—often only a month—and no evaluation of the comparative cost of the drug or the side-effects profile.

Consider, for a moment, a comparison of the percentage of the health care dollar spent on medications by a policy decision not to use tricyclic antidepressant medications because there are newer and "safer" drugs on the market. There is no difference in the efficacy of these newer drugs; that is, they are not superior in treating depression, and they are an order of magnitude more expensive. They are safer in the context that tricyclics are more lethal when used to overdose and some tricyclics are associated with higher rates of patients who have acute myocardial infarctions (heart attacks). However, the side-effects profile of these newer selective serotonin reuptake inhibitor (SSRI) medications have a 33% side-effect rate of sexual dysfunction, which leads to poor compliance. The point is that hundreds of millions of dollars are used inefficiently because clinicians have difficulty incorporating a cost/benefit assessment into their clinical decision making, which depletes precious health care resources.

Our medical technology is considered to be the best in the world. However, its development has been extremely expensive because of the lack of planning and regulation. Most of us have not learned how to use it effectively and efficiently in clinical practice. There are no controls over how many high-tech devices such as computed tomography (CT) or magnetic resonance imaging (MRI) machines there are in one geographic area. This is one major category where our clinical resources would have been better utilized by using a certificate-of-need rationale and *clinical protocols* to save those precious resources for better matched treatment interventions (Eisenberg, 1986). One premise involved with a certificate of need is that one must justify how efficiently a very costly machine will be used based on the needs of a given population to be served. If that subset of the population who will require these services is not large enough to maximize the use of the machine, then it is more appropriate to share another one that is more efficient. By having too many machines in one geographic area, costs per evaluation are increased to cover the basic expense of the machine, creating a situation where the cost of the procedure is too high for many of those who might appropriately benefit from it. This situation also creates double jeopardy by tempting clinicians to overutilize the technique in cases for which it has not been demonstrated to be effective. For example, CT scans dramatically improve the treatment of head injuries, but this procedure is misused in the investigation of headaches (Starr, 1982).

Clinical protocols will provide the road map for consistency and reliability in the way health care services are delivered. They are the prototype in the continuous refinement of matching patient need with the best service(s) to be delivered. Protocols and guidelines have been developed by a number of organizations including the American Psychiatric Association (Mattson, 1992), the Agency for Healthcare Policy and Research (Depression Guideline Panel, 1993), and the Institute of Medicine (Field & Lohr, 1990) and are based on national standards.

MANAGED CARE

Managed care (MC) is here to stay. It is an encompassing term used to define ways of delivering, managing and evaluating clinical services. The forms of managed care will change, but the principles such as service quality, clinical effectiveness, and efficiencies that have withstood the test of time will remain. The first generation of managed care was born in 1929, with the establishment of the Ross-Loos Clinic as the first health maintenance organization (HMO). Group Health Association, based in Washington, D.C., was founded in 1937 (Health Insurance Association of America, 1994). However the percentage of people who selected this coordinated prepaid group-practice approach to care was small during the following decades until it exploded in the early 1980s.

We are in our fourth generation of MC, called *behavioral health carveouts*, which provide *fourth-party*, *quality management* of care. This model blossomed in the late 1980s. *Behavioral carveout* is a term used to describe a model of care and management that separates out the provision and payment of mental health and chemical dependence services from medical-surgical services. The *fourth party* is defined as the clinical management organization, that component which reviews care for *medical necessity* but often is different from the direct deliverer of clinical services to patients (Mattson, 1992). The essential elements of this model type include a *network* of clinicians who provide services to patients, who are beneficiaries or members of a health plan. Clinicians from the four core disciplines of psychiatry, psychiatric nursing, psychology, and social work are invited to join a network *privileging*. There is a formal structure in the managed care organization designed to evaluate the ongoing quality of the clinical and other services provided by clinicians. These skills are measured in a number of ways, such as comparing clinicians' practice patterns with one another, evaluating individual clinical care, asking patients for feedback, and assessing clinical outcomes. This network model permits managed care organizations to evaluate the quality of care provided to patients, using different tools of measurement to consider patient outcomes. Network providers are given clinical protocols and comparative information from other clinicians on their own practice patterns. One goal is to provide quality care to optimize the health status of patients. Clinical quality is measured by assessing patient outcomes. Clinicians enhance their care by continuously improving the services they provide. Given the focus on quality for our network clinicians, there are monetary savings for patients who select a clinician from their health plans' networks. It costs more for members to select clinicians who are not in the network. Today, some element of MC principles is incorporated in all health care that is not paid fully and directly by the patient, that is, which involves a third-party payor.

Perhaps the greatest dilemma in dealing with the paradigm shift of MC is that these new demands do not reflect the way we were taught to be clinicans. Nor does this MC reality match our expectations of being our own bosses. We have invested a great deal of resources and made tremendous sacrifices in time, expenditures, and lost revenue to master clinical skills so that we may call ourselves clinicians (Schwabb, 1994). No one has taught us how to do a comparative analysis of one treatment over another, or how to utilize resources as if they were our own, or that "less" and "more" do not necessarily equal "optimal" services (Austad & Berman, 1991). An example of "more" not equaling "optimal" is the 1980s example of hospitalizing a chemically dependent person for 28 days to complete an inpatient program. The overall results were disastrous, since most of these programs did not provide aftercare to deal with the issues of craving and being exposed to one's real environment after discharge. Outpatient programs designed with these issues in mind had much better rates for patients maintaining sobriety or staying drug free. By evaluating the differences in these programs, clinicians increase their ability to choose appropriate services for their patients. The outcome is better patient care, and in this example, at great savings to make available to the health care pool of resources.

Another issue—especially for nonphysician *behavioral health clinicians*—is that a clinician's orientation may not be based on a medical or public health model but rather on a psychological one. Therefore, the whole person, including a person's physical well-being, has not been considered in terms of the now required biopsychosocial model. This gap creates problems for the client/patient as well as the clinician, since it has been well demonstrated (Jones & Vischi, 1979; Manning et al., 1986) that taking a holistic approach in a patient's assessment and treatment has demonstrably improved her or his health status. This approach has become the driving force in maximizing availability for clinical services using health care dollars. Example: if a woman comes into treatment and says that she is depressed but the therapist does not elicit that she is involved in a violent home situation, then the therapist has not put this patient in the context of her environment. Therefore, the clinician will not be able to develop a quality treatment intervention that will meet this patient's needs.

Some may consider MC to be a powerful system, demanding that we think and work in a different way "or else." The "or else" is a decreased income and the need to learn very different skills at a time when we thought we had completed that major phase of our education and development of our work role. How did this happen? Several converging forces that took root in the early 1980s suggest why the current fourth-party model of MC companies flourishes with such intensity.

SPIRALING COSTS

A major issue that increasingly concerned corporations and smaller businesses was that the costs of their share of payment for their employees' health benefits were spiraling out of control at rates that were two to four times the rate of inflation per year. The rise in employer spending on health benefits increased 163% between 1970 and 1989 (15.6% per year), compared with 30% for retirement benefits over the same 20 years, resulting in stagnating real take-home pay for employees (Starr, 1994). Employer health-benefit payout for employees was the major category that was out of control. When behavioral health care costs were compared with costs for other medical care, the rates of increase for behavioral health care were much higher. Remember the 28-day mandated inpatient chemical dependence treatment strategy of the 1980s? The rationale for states to mandate care was to ensure that clinical services were available to patients in need. However, this policy of mandating 28 days of inpatient care (rather than setting some patient outcome measures) utilized tremendous resources, paying for expensive bed days, but it did not have a major impact on recidivism. Thus, this strategy alone utilized tremendous resources with little impact on improved health status (Yahr, 1988; Saxe & Goodman, 1988).

For many small employers, who as a group employ a majority of people in this country, this health-benefit expense became so great that 13% have eliminated health benefits (1991) and another 30% are expected to be forced to drop health benefits in the future if there are no changes in dealing with health care (Bureau of Labor Statistics, 1991).

This explosion in costs caught the attention of chief executive officers and managers, since the end result, if the trend were not stopped, would be bankruptcy, job loss, loss of revenue for investors, recession, and elimination of health benefits. Therefore they hurriedly and unexpertly developed a series of strategies to hold the line and stop the hemorrhaging of their bottom lines.

A little-known fact in clinical circles is that it is employers, not the third-party insurance companies, who offer the types of benefits from which their employees may select. Basically, the 1980s have been a nightmare for the benefit managers of corporations who had to come up with benefit designs that would not cause companies to go bankrupt. These experiments are what patients and clinicians are dealing with now: lifetime caps of dollar amounts paid out for behavioral health care, lifetime number of covered hospitalizations, dramatic decreases in the number of paid outpatient sessions, fourth-party MC companies obliged to preauthorize care that is considered effective and efficient, and so on. This has resulted in outraged patients and clinicians who do not understand the process.

Clinicians are experiencing the movement from what was once a private-practice model of health care into a public health model in which the payors of care take a very active interest in the outcome and costs of treatment delivered. Another result is that benefit managers have learned that the bottom line must incorporate quality of care, because poor quality is more expensive. A third development is that MC companies have learned more about how to manage quality of care and services. Consider the evolution from retrospective individual case review to concurrent review. Retrospective review is a paper-documented review of care that is complete; therefore there is no possibility of intervening in that particular treatment episode except for making a decision about payment of services. Concurrent review of care occurs while a patient is being treated. Therefore there is opportunity for a clinical consultation to alter the course of treatment. In the earlier example of a woman in treatment for depression, her therapist was unaware that the patient was currently in a violent situation at home. A consultation could occur between the therapist and the clinician in the managed care company to incorporate this very important piece of information, which would then change the treatment plan to work for a better outcome.

This critical influence of managed care would not be so great if citizens paid for their health care out of pocket. Indeed, it would be a private affair. However, the citizens of this country believe that health care needs to be subsidized for everyone to allow earlier intervention and better health status and to prevent personal bankruptcy due to illness in the family. At the moment, despite the United States' world leadership in health care technology, something is seriously wrong when it ranks eleventh in the world based on the health status of its citizens (U.S. Commerce Department, 1993). Some 17% of its mostly employed citizens are without health care coverage, which is the world's most expensive health care by margins of other major nations' entire gross national products (Reinhardt, 1990).

Another major trend in the 1980s that spawned MC companies was that large companies chose to self-insure using provisions from the employee retirement income security act (ERISA) of 1974, rather than using third parties as payors, in order to gain greater control in managing health resources and greater freedom from state regulations. For example, the furor over lack of chemical dependence (CD) coverage in many health benefit plans in the mid-1980s resulted in state legislation mandating that, for example, all citizens living in a particular state were entitled to 60 days of inpatient CD care (Health Insurance Association of America, 1989). Although this state law for benefit coverage had great intentions to protect and provide care for those needing treatment, the result was that many people were hospitalized for 30 or 60 days with no/few provisions for transition to home and work, which resulted in tremendous relapse rates and poor outcomes as well as great expense and waste of resources. Since the large corporations did not have to comply with such regulations, this left a smaller base over which to spread the costs.

INCREASED RATES AND SEVERITY OF ILLNESS

The 1980s also brought tripled suicide rates for adolescents, a national drug epidemic, and dramatic increases in rates of major depression and violence

(U.S. Commerce Department, 1993; Handgun Control Inc., 1992). Treating people with major depression and bipolar disorders has become much more complex, requiring intricate pharmacologic and other therapeutic interventions. Part of the reason is found in the genetic contribution to major depression. As researchers further refine major depression, it has been determined that part of the genetic code, deoxyribonucleic acid sequences called triplet repeats, have become unstable, that is, should not form this way and promote greater severity of illness in patients with this sequencing. This is just one of many intricacies of depression (Depaulo, 1994).

A major response to the increased numbers of people developing illness was a mushrooming of free-standing psychiatric and chemical dependence facilities throughout the nation. These hospitals were often built without requiring a certificate-of-need (CON) assessment to demonstrate that these beds were necessary for a particular community. Occupancy rates fell to an all-time low (15 to 30%), resulting in cost shifting to the public sector, so that governments were paying for private-sector greed and poor fiscal responsibility and management (Reinhardt, 1990; Wilensky, 1984). Behavioral health care continued to demonstrate its differences from the rest of medicine when it claimed that it was more of a healing art than a science and stayed out of the first round of governmental attempts to quantify the resources needed to treat a particular disorder. This classification of illnesses paired with the quantification of resources needed to appropriately treat is called diagnostic related groups (DRGs) and has been used in the medical-surgical clinical specialties except for psychiatry since the early 1980s (Wennberg et al., 1984).

MANAGED CARE PRINCIPLES

Health maintenance organizations continued with their mission to provide quality health care delivered efficiently, accessed equally by all their subscribers. An essential component for these organizations, in assessing whether care is provided consistently and effectively, is the ability to evaluate clinical information. Electronic information systems continue to increase their powerful role as a tool that not only has transformed our society but is essential to the refinement of analyses needed to establish whether specific treatments and patient outcomes are consistent, reliable, and valid. Because HMOs are designed around multidisciplinary group practice models and systems of care concepts, they are able to create clinician, patient, and member databases to review how care is delivered, at what cost, and for which outcomes. It is these principles that have survived into the 1990s and have become essential requirements for all clinical practice.

Currently, managed care companies carve out behavioral health interventions and management; they seek to develop a partnership with clinicians who understand this paradigm shift in health care. Clinicians who do not comprehend this process have been unable to distinguish the differences in clinical practices between themselves and their managed care colleagues; they therefore feel left out.

PUBLIC HEALTH APPROACH

Although public health principles and information have been around for a century, this model is finally reaching a critical mass and surpassing the traditional medical model. It is clear that early intervention, at an earlier stage in the process of disease, costs less and leads to better outcomes. Educating people to incorporate good eating and exercise habits, eliminate nicotine, limit alcohol, maintain adequate rest, and follow vaccination protocols would dramatically slash the costs of providing health care services. Our tool of instant communication and information will better provide accurate health information to allow consumers to make better-informed choices about health services. Unless taken as additional areas of interest and training, none of the traditional four core disciplines of psychiatry, psychology, psychiatric nursing, and social work have integrated much knowledge and experience from the public health approach. Coordinated care goes along with this model. This contrasts with the traditional, independent, solo-practice fee-for-service approach.

EFFECTIVENESS OF SERVICES

How do we measure effectiveness? There are several ways to approach this issue. One is for clinicians to compare the treatments we provide to our patients. We will find some variance in our results that has to do with our uneven application of our services. Another approach is to compare our treatment with that of our colleagues' treatment of similar patients with the same severity of illness. Another is to compare our treatments with the national standards. All of these methods are useful in keeping ourselves up-to-date on current treatment and evaluation (Wennberg, 1985; Winickoff et al., 1984).

WHAT WILL OUR PRACTICE LOOK LIKE?

The way we deliver services will look and feel totally different. The themes are coordinated care, optimal treatment, and outcome evaluation. Very refined services are being matched to meet very specific treatment needs, updated on line, in a continuous fashion so that there is a seamless and timely relationship between scientific findings and their implementation in clinical practice (Beller, 1994).

If you are still in solo practice, it will be essential to consider electronic linkage with systems that provide state-of-the-art practice guidelines. These guidelines will describe best practices, clinical decision trees, or essential elements of care to be considered as a quality intervention for a particular treatment. It will also be critical to be linked up with other clinicians who provide other kinds of clinical services. Examples of integrative care include working with psychiatrists, and/or experts in the areas of child care, such as pediatricians, or family care, such as family practitioners, or specialists in women's health.

We need to continuously master information systems to make them work for us. We will be expected to keep abreast of our field, which has experienced incredible changes in very brief periods of time. Also, we will be expected to be part of a network of colleagues so that a full-service delivery system can be provided by calling just one person in this network. This is the concept of one-stop shopping in taking care of our health.

WHAT TOOLS WILL WE NEED?

My vision is that we will need a method to keep pace with new clinical information plus a way to use information systems to assist us in standardizing our information and keeping it reliable and consistent. We will need to tap into a system that identifies state-of-the-art clinical practice parameters. We will need new skills, such as a proficiency in the use of information systems and public-health concepts and practices, as well as knowledge and experience of new treatment findings and practices.

WHY THIS IS A CHALLENGING AND REWARDING TIME TO BE A CLINICIAN

Science and technology are hurtling us through life at warp speed. And it appears that those of us in the behavioral health field are having perhaps the greatest difficulty in adaptation. The naysayers are vocal in expressing their fear of change, which seems to be a resonant response when there is any major societal upheaval. Sameness is comforting when the future seems so different.

I often think of this period and wonder how much our response to its impact is similar to the farmers' response to the industrial revolution. Cultural transformation changes our lives so much! A major difference between the industrial and technology revolutions and the changes of today is the incredible speed driving this current epoch. Our vast knowledge base in human behavior grows exponentially, seemingly at the speed of light. And we clinicians have learned merely an outline and not the full text that puts life and behavior into focus. We, who are called experts in the psychology of life, are expected to know how to care for those who come to us for help, direction, guidance, and learning.

Despite the fact that our skills and techniques are quickly becoming outmoded, our mission remains the same.

Many view this new paradigm as progress. It is. This is a time of great opportunity, exploration, and learning. The excitement comes with the experience of being on the cutting edge and knowing that one is making a difference.

REFERENCES

Austad, C. S., & Berman, W. H. (Eds.) (1991). *Psychotherapy in managed health-care: The optimal use of time and resources*. Washington, DC: American Psychological Association.

Beller, S. E. (1994). A comprehensive-integrated electronic information network system for cost-control and continuous quality improvement of mental health-care. In *Navigating reform: HMOs and managed care in a time of transition*, (pp. 345–375). Washington, DC: Group Health Association of America.

Borus, J. F., Olendski, M. C., Kessler, L., et al. (1985). The offset effect of mental health treatment on ambulatory medical care utilization and charges. *Archives of General Psychiatry*, 42:573–580.

Bunch, B., & Hellemans, A. (Eds.) (1994). *The timetables of technology*. New York: Simon & Schuster.

Bureau of Labor Statistics. (1991). Washington, DC: U.S. Department of Labor.

Depaulo, R. J. (1994). Presentation of research findings. Presented at the Canadian Psychiatric Association Annual Meeting, Ottawa.

Depression Guideline Panel (1993). *Clinical practice guideline #5: Depression in primary care*. Three volumes. Agency for Health Care Policy and Research #93-0550. Rockville, M.D.: Department of Health and Human Services/Public Health Service/Agency for Health Care Policy and Research.

Detsky, A. S., Nagalie, G. N., & Krahn, M. D. (1994). Clinical decision analysis. *Annals of the Royal College of Physicians and Surgeons of Canada, 27*, 3:157–159.

Eisenberg, J. M. (1986). *Doctors' decisions and the cost of medical care*. Ann Arbor, Michigan: Health Administration Press Perspectives.

Field, M. J., & Lohr, K. N., (Eds.) (1990). *Clinical Practice Guidelines*. Institute of Medicine. Washington, DC: National Academy Press.

Employee Retirement Income Security Act (ERISA) (1974).

Gray, B. H., & Field, M. J. (Eds.) (1989). *Controlling costs and changing patient care?* Institute of Medicine. Washington, DC: National Academy Press.

Handgun Control Inc. (1992). Washington, DC.

Health Insurance Association of America. (1994). *Source book of health insurance data 1993.* Washington, DC: Health Insurance Association of America.

———, (1989). *On health insurance issues, state mandated benefits.*

Hoeper, E. W., & Nyca, G. R. (1981). Utilization and cost of mental healthcare when integrated in a healthcare system. *Journal of Psychiatric Treatments and Evaluation, 3,* 117–226.

Jones, K. R., & Vischi, T. R. (1979). Impact of alcohol, drug abuse and mental health treatment on medical utilization: A review of the literature. *Medical Care, 17* (supplement), 1–82.

Kuhn, T. S. (1970). *The structure of scientific revolutions* (second edition). Chicago: University of Chicago Press.

Manning, W. G., Wells, K. B., & Benjamin, B. (1986). *Use of outpatient mental healthcare: Trial of a prepaid group practice versus fee for service.* Santa Monica, CA: Rand Corporation.

Mattson, M. R. (Ed.) (1992). *Manual of psychiatric quality assurance.* Washington, DC: American Psychiatric Press.

101st Congress, Public Law 101, July 25. (1989). *The decade of the brain.* Washington, DC: U.S. Joint House/Senate Resolution.

Reinhardt, U. E. (1990). *Providing access to healthcare and controlling costs: Approach abroad, options for the United States.* Ethics of science lecture. Greater Baltimore Medical Center. 25th Anniversary National Conference, Baltimore MD.

Saxe, L., & Goodman, L. (1988). *The effect of outpatient versus inpatient chemical dependence treatment.* Revised internal document. Congress of the United States Office of Technology Assessment.

Schwabb, E. (1994). Clinical inservice, unpublished. Empire Mental Health Choice, Empire Blue Cross/Blue Shield. New York, N.Y.

Starr, P. (1994). *The logic of healthcare reform.* New York: Whittle.

——— (1982). *The social transformation of American medicine.* New York: Basic Books.

Tyler, M. (1994). Personal communication.

U.S. Commerce Department, Census Bureau. (1993). *Statistical abstracts,* 113.

Vandenbos, G., & Deleon, H. H. (1988). The use of psychotherapy to improve physical health. *Psychotherapy: Theory, research, and practice, 25:* 3, 335–343.

Wennberg, J. E. (1985). On patient need, equity, supplier induced demand and the need to assess the outcome of common medical practices. *Medical Care, 23:* 5, 512–520.

———, McPherson, K., & Caper, P. (1984). Will payment based on diagnosis related groups control hospital costs? *New England Journal of Medicine, 311:* 5, 295–300.

Wilensky, G. O. (1984). Solving uncompensated care. *Health Affairs* (winter).

Winickoff, R. N., Coltin, K. L., Morgan, M. M., et al. (1984). Improving physician performance through peer comparison feedback. *Medicare Care*, 22: 6, 527–534.

Yahr, H. T. (1988). A national comparison of public and private sector alcoholism treatment delivery system characteristics. *Journal of Studies in Alcohol*, 49: 3, 233–239.

CHAPTER 2

The Mechanics of Developing a Successful Behavioral Group Practice for Managed Care: How to Survive in the Competitive Field of Mental Health Practice

Sidney H. Grossberg

A BRIEF HISTORY

Nearly two decades ago, my present partner (a psychiatrist) and I (a university teacher and social worker) decided to form a multidisciplinary group practice. Fortunately for us, it was an auspicious time in Michigan to start a group practice. The auto companies and the UAW had just negotiated a contract with Blue Cross/Blue Shield to provide mental health benefits for auto employees, and what they wanted were multidisciplinary clinics meeting specific criteria for staffing, clinical procedures, and record keeping. These clinics would then be accredited as outpatient psychiatric clinics or "OPCs."

After meeting these criteria, we decided to go after as many other national and state accreditations as possible, such as Joint Commission on Accreditation of Healthcare Organizations (JCAHO), State of Michigan Office of Substance Abuse Services, and the Commission on Accreditation of Rehabilitative Facilities (CARF°). We are licensed by the state of Michigan as a substance abuse provider. It is always good to have a license, not just an accreditation, because many managed care and insurance companies look for them, believing that licenses are protection against malpractice judgments. When you get accreditations, you are able to use this achievement as a marketing tool.

We began as a group of three; today we number over 75 therapists augmented by three contracted psychiatrists, and we are still growing. Not being businessmen, we had to learn how to convert intuition into profitable, ethical professional strategies.

What follows here is a basic primer for developing and operating a successful group practice for managed care. It is based on 23 years of personal experience. A successfully operating group practice is not unlike a smooth-running machine. Assembly, manufacture, and maintenance may require tinkerings and tuneups, but if all the parts are properly placed in the beginning—and, of course, kept properly oiled—utility and quality are virtually guaranteed!

THE BASICS: INCORPORATION AND ACCREDITATION

Many practitioners who consult with me have already formed small group practices. However, for those readers who have yet to do so, let us begin with the basic mechanics.

The first step is to hire an attorney to incorporate your practice according to the laws of your state, as each state's laws are unique. The attorney will draw up articles of incorporation or partnership and see to it that each owner receives stock certificates in the corporation. If you decide to begin as a simple partnership, be aware that this may leave you personally responsible for the actions of your partners.

You can begin as a "C" corporation (a normal business corporation) or as a "Subchapter S" corporation (in which income or losses flow directly through to the owner's personal tax returns); each has different tax ramifications. We started out as a "Sub S" because we expected to lose money for the first 3 years and wished to have the losses flow through to our personal income and to limit our potential losses to the initial capital invested

---

°CARF is located in Tucson, AZ, and I recommend it highly as it is friendly to private-practice rehabilitation facilities.

in the corporation. What we wanted was a simple incorporation so that we could do business but not lose our homes and other assets should the business go bankrupt. In some states, there is a new entity called an "LLC" or limited liability corporation, that combines the best of the above. Any good attorney can provide an inexpensive "canned" articles of incorporation package that conforms to state requirements. This would also be the time to select a name and clear it with the "assumed names division" in your state. Filing your name with the state guarantees that no other party can use it. Costs can increase substantially if you begin to formulate a buyout agreement between partners, a pension or profit-sharing plan, or a medical reimbursement plan. A buyout plan is needed if one partner dies, wants to retire or leave, or is permanently disabled. It is better to have a signed agreement as to how a buyout will be carried out and to be financed before any such occurrence. Otherwise a business partner's surviving spouse, children, or estate can sue for fair compensation and tie up the corporation in court for a prolonged period of time. There are legal costs for writing such plans. There are also the costs of paying off the estate of a deceased partner plus the cost of replacing that partner. Often such plans can be funded by life or disability insurance.

The next step is to select an accountant who will work out payroll, keep you apprised of taxes and payments, and help to prepare and file federal, state, and local corporation and tax reports. The accountant can even help to set up a financial report so that you can determine monthly costs and expenses.

The final step is to purchase shares in the corporation and set up an office. You sign a lease for 1 or 2 years (short-term leases are more costly), hire a secretary (preferable to an answering machine), print up business cards, and—as soon as it is affordable—prepare an inexpensive brochure to use for marketing, one that can be upgraded as the practice grows.

THE "BEST": SELECTING A STAFF

It has been our philosophy that if we hire the best possible people, referrals will then follow. So the "kingpin" is always to go after the best. Find the most knowledgeable and experienced therapists you can, representing a spectrum of modalities. Make sure you have child and adolescent therapists, substance abuse therapists, and family therapists, and that you hire people who give good, intensive treatment, whether it be long or short term. We preferred our staff to have at least 5 years past their master's degree, be it in psychology or social work. As we expanded, so many different kinds of cases came to us that, in effect, we turned into a kind of traditional family service agency with an array of credentialed practitioners who could diagnose and treat within their areas of expertise. As to how we select and evaluate our staff: We have a credentialing committee that looks over new or potential hirees' licenses, each therapist's certificate or malpractice insurance, and university transcripts; the committee also conducts a re-credentialing update every 2 years (thereby satisfying CARF, JCAHO, and insurance and managed care companies' demands for quality assurance). We also utilize a company called Credential Check, located in Farmington Hills, Michigan, that reviews the credentials of applicants.

By design, we selected many part-time therapists who had specific areas of expertise, although we never advertised them as such. Not only was this a way to generate referrals from their colleagues but, more importantly, it enabled us to serve a large number of patients with a host of different mental health and substance abuse problems. Our clients came from all strata of society, including some on Medicaid and Medicare who required a gamut of services ranging from substance abuse treatment to traditional, psychoanalytically oriented psychotherapy.

Pragmatically speaking, we found it advisable to avoid therapists who were into new and vague types of therapy. Trendy therapists are likely to commit malpractice; therefore, a clinic that hires them runs the risk of being sued and out of business very, very fast. In a course I teach at Smith College, entitled "Avoiding Malpractice," I stress that therapists must understand what constitutes malpractice and that they must practice by the prevailing community standards. Good solid psychotherapy with an accompanying understanding of transference and countertransference issues and well-documented records help to avoid malpractice suits. However, since everyone is potentially liable, we have liability insurance for the company itself, its owners, and the board of directors, and we require every therapist to have his or her own malpractice insurance as well.

Our therapists are independent contractors who also work elsewhere and who are paid for their services when the fees are collected. In addition, we contract with the three psychiatrists on an hourly basis. If the patient does not pay, the therapist does not get paid; and we, as risk sharers, also do not get paid. It is best to consult with an attorney who will provide criteria for independent contractors and then set up a contract accordingly; potential problems with the IRS are thus avoided.

The clinic has secretaries, receptionists, an answering service, rooms, referrals, billings, and marketing, as well as educational and supervision opportunities. Our therapists have the opportunity to accept or refuse referrals and slowly, even those who were most opposed to treating managed care patients have come around. Each month the secretaries circulate a list to all therapists asking how many hours they have currently and how many more hours they want.

We assist therapists by helping them to translate their recorded case notes into specific behavioral terms. For example, instead of recording that a patient is "depressed," we teach therapists to state "patient is tired all the time" or "patient can't sleep."

A practice grows when there are therapists available to see patients at the times *they* need or the times they are able to be seen. This is especially true in these uneasy economic times when employees risk losing their jobs if they take too much time off from work. A clinic has to have the capability of offering a variety of hours, with no waiting list, so that people can be seen the very day or within the week that they call. I should add that every company interested in doing business with us wants to know if we maintain a 24-hour line. We do. We instruct the 24-hour answering service that on-going patients who need to talk to their therapists have 24-hour coverage. If the caller has never been seen before, we have the answering service ask if the problem can wait until morning. If the answer is no, the service provides a list of hospitals. On the other hand, we have secretarial coverage from 8 A.M. to 10 P.M. Monday through Thursday and 8 A.M. to 6 P.M. on Fridays and until 5 P.M. on Saturday. Therapists also see patients after regular office hours, including Sundays.

The number of group practices are increasing dramatically and it is widely accepted that individual clinicians are going to have problems getting referrals during this period of health care reform. Managed care companies are looking for group practices.

For the most part, managed care companies *prefer* to deal with group practices. Rather than having to search through their computer database for a therapist in a specific geographic location who can work with a specific age group, with a specific problem at specified times during the week, the managed care company can do all this at once by referring to a group practice. The practice contact person must then match the client with the appropriate therapist. The group practice one-stop shopping is an excellent selling point to managed care companies.

Some managed care companies use the anchor group concept. A large group in a specific geographic area handles all emergency referrals and must triage them to help keep referrals in the least restrictive care possible. Only after the triage effort can the anchor group allow hospitalization.

If less restrictive care is called for or if referral to another resource is necessary, this can be done by the anchor group. Many managed care companies are even giving anchor groups capitation contracts to provide services for all potential plan enrollees in an area.

Managed care and insurance companies usually look for the following qualifications in a group practice, as aptly put by the Institute for Behavioral Health Care membership criteria for their Council of Behavioral

Group Practices:

- Full economic and operational integration
- Professional administration
- Computerized management and information systems
- Strong commitment to managed behavioral health care services
- Ten or more full-time behavioral health practitioners
- Psychiatrists fully integrated into practice
- 24-hour access
- Quality assurance programs
- Care management and continuity of care systems

They also want one federal employee identification number to be used for tax purposes.

One of the major advantages of this type of a group practice is that it generates referrals. For example, if you get a marriage case and a therapist prefers not to see the couple together, the group practice concept generates interclinic referrals. Now there are two referrals instead of just one.

In my consultations across the country on how to start and develop group practices and make them grow, I stress that it can be a difficult process unless done properly, economically, legally, and ethically. An additional group practice benefit is that insurance companies such as Blue Cross will reimburse for psychotherapy services because it is an interdisciplinary effort. The key words with insurance companies are *medical necessity*. Treatment for *medical conditions requiring psychotherapy* is reimbursed. You should always be cognizant of this because the insurance companies are. When we first started out, we geared ourselves to the patients and to insurance companies. Now we gear ourselves also to managed care companies. Organizing your clinic as a multidisciplinary setting with a medical person in charge is almost a practical necessity, because treatment in that kind of setting is what companies want.

THE "OIL": OPTIMUM WORKING CONDITIONS

If you want a clinic to grow, you must have satisfied staff members—and, in addition to payment, people want good working conditions. Now you can subsume everything under good working conditions, including growth and development, in-service training, and attractive offices. We have done just that by establishing committees to address every aspect of clinic functioning. We have a hiring committee of clinicians to interview new staff applicants and make recommendations to the chief executive officer as to whether they should be accepted to work at the clinic; a credentialing committee, which sees that continued education is up to date; a staff meeting administrating committee that sets meeting agendas; an education committee that selects speakers; and a safety committee in accord with the JCAHO and CARF standards of safety. We also have an orientation committee whose chairperson conducts a 2-hour session with each new staff member to go over our staff manual, explain billing and record-keeping procedures, and literally provide the new contractor with the keys to the building. There is even a "good and welfare" committee that selects and sends out gifts when staff members give birth, celebrate an anniversary, fall ill, or are bereaved. There is a marketing committee that helps to develop and implement our marketing plan.

In part because it makes sense and in part because it is required by Blue Cross/Blue Shield of Michigan, CARF, and managed care companies, our clinic developed a Utilization Review Quality Assurance Committee consisting of our psychiatrist-owner, at least one fully licensed psychologist, the social work clinical director, and three additional staff members. On a bimonthly basis, this committee reviews approximately 20% of all of our cases regarding appropriate staff assignment, diagnosis and treatment plans, supportive services, duration of treatment, continuity of treatment planning and discharge, as well as whether patients' records are complete and up to date. The therapists receive feedback on every case reviewed, and we request a reply that is then checked over by one of the committee members. In addition, we have an internal closing audit to ensure that records are dictated and current, that there is an intake and a quarterly summary, and that all of the progress notes are documented. It is essential that there be a system in place to make certain that every service provided is documented and medically necessary. Otherwise, there is the danger that money will be reclaimed by insurance or managed care companies, and the patient's integral right to good and continuous care will be jeopardized.

At our clinic, far and away the most powerful committee is the Room Committee, whose task it is to equitably fit 75 therapists into 36 offices. All room requests go through the Room Committee, which, being composed of colleagues and peers, is accepted as the legitimate, ultimate authority. Moreover, such a system creates maximum office utilization and demonstrates cost-efficiency to managed care and insurance companies. In addition, we have instituted a special Policy and Problems Committee and a Retrospective Study Committee that conducts the research studies required by Blue Cross and the managed care companies.

We try to provide at least one ongoing seminar for staff at all times. The continuing education we provide can also be used for recredentialing, thereby satisfying CARF, JCAHO, and managed care requirements for quality assurance.

THE "DRIVE": MARKETING AND PUBLIC RELATIONS

If you want your practice to grow, you absolutely must market. There just was not enough time to promote ourselves to all of the growing number of managed care companies. The solution was to create a marketing committee composed primarily of our more aggressive, community-active therapists. They make initial forays into the community (whereas I do the basic marketing), following up on companies that have expressed an interest in our services. I feed "leads" to the committee chairperson, who then assigns them to committee members. A helpful source for contacts, I have found, is the Institute for Behavioral Health Care Conference, where you can interact in person with companies. Most of these companies are besieged by as many as 1000 requests a week and would not know you from Adam if you contacted them initially by telephone and had not met them at the conference.

Our clinic has achieved success as much by intuition as by organized planning. Our clinic guidelines are fairness, honesty, and quality. Notwithstanding, satisfying managed care company guidelines for referrals has led me to develop a more formalized marketing–management system. The messages that these marketing stratagems communicate to the community are that our clinic offers *versatility of services*; *quality staff*; *immediate appointments*—daytime, evening, and weekend; *convenient location*; *accreditations*; and *reimbursement by insurance plans*.

The market plan is to first analyze the marketplace, your own capacities, your fellow providers, and the general environment; then develop a plan of action, implement it, and evaluate. Since *Counseling Associates* is a private, for-profit organization, the objectives are as follow:

1. Continuously increase the number of referrals coming into the clinic as measured by the number of referrals that increase each year.
2. Increase the number of service units (i.e., interview sessions) as measured by the yearly increase in interviews.
3. Employ the most experienced and highly qualified clinicians as measured by the percentage of staff with a master's, Ph.D., or M.D. degree and board certified diplomates in social work.
4. Provide consumer satisfaction (through the alleviation of distress and symptomatology) as measured by outcomes surveys and consumer satisfaction studies.

Whenever a case is terminated at our clinic, the patient is given a consumer satisfaction questionnaire that includes such questions as: "Has the quality of your life improved at work? In your social relationships? How was your ease of entry into the clinic? Were you easily able to find our location? Was the receptionist courteous and polite? Were there are billing problems?"

An excellent and powerful, yet inexpensive outcome software system is the mental health/substance abuse version of the Beaumont Outcome Software System.*

My philosophy is that every referral helps, and if you do not go after referrals, you are going to be locked out and eventually you will not have any patients at all. I market according to this philosophy. For example, I get a copy of every referral that comes to the clinic and then send the therapist a pretyped slip that says, "Could you please contact 'X' and thank him or her for making the referral to us." This not only provides feedback to the referral source but also reinforces awareness of our clinic.

I subscribe to most magazines and journals in the field of mental health and human relations benefits, and every time I spy a company (employee assistance programs, insurance, health maintenance organizations, and preferred provider organizations) that we do not have a contract with, I either call or give the name to my marketing committee to contact, saying, "We are a very large outpatient psychiatric clinic in the Detroit area staffed with 75 therapists who can handle immediate appointments in substance abuse, posttraumatic stress syndrome, and so on. Do you have any contracts in the Detroit area? If so, we would like to be your exclusive provider in the area." Here it is helpful to have an already developed brochure to send for their perusal, in which you emphasize the versatility of your group.

Target small- to medium-sized companies as well, looking for those with insurance that will reimburse your clinic. And do not forget school systems that might like to initiate an employee-assistance program. We have posters telling about our services and distribute them to school systems for posting in staff rooms. The posters say: "For confidential help regarding family problems, child and adolescent problems, and so on, contact Counseling Associates." We have developed a program of seminars and speakers and mailed out a listing of these events to school systems and family service agencies. Whether you are just starting out or are trying to grow, survey your staff as to what they feel they can lecture about. Make up your own list and mail it to generate interest, which in turn leads to referrals.

---

*Sidney Grossberg, Richard Merson, Michael Rolnick, & Fred Weiner. (1995) *Beaumont Outcome Software System: Mental Health Version*. Michigan: Parrot Software.

A source of referrals for us has been cost-effective advertisements in the Yellow Pages. We designed a very professional looking ad and were the first group to use a large ad rather than just our name. Our referrals increased for the year, and we had more money to run even bigger (but still tasteful) ads and to advertise in more places. We inserted our ad under "Psychologists," "Marriage Counselors," "Substance Abuse," "Social Work," and "Mental Health Centers." As our referrals grew, we determined where our patients were coming from and refined the placement of the ads.

Our clinic maintains interagency agreements with mental health hospitals, substance abuse hospitals, and a vocational service agency as well. We have surrounded ourselves with a complete mental health system, and we use this as a marketing tool.

We have also established a Community Advisory Board that functions as our eyes and ears to the community at large, provides referrals, and, in effect, facilitates accreditations, as some companies require a community advisory board, and CARF routinely inquires if a clinic is active in the community. Currently, we have a union person on the board, an insurance executive, the head of a department at a major Detroit area hospital, a pediatrician, a business-person, and a psychiatrist. We review our staff selection and policies with them, and they help us to assess what the community needs. Of particular help is that they brainstorm with us and, in the process, generate some excellent advice on business practices.

When mental health practitioners from around the country call me to help them negotiate through the maze of managed health care, my consultation consists of much of the material in this chapter. My foremost advice is to form or join a group practice in order to survive the changes in mental health care.

CHAPTER 3

Case Management and Review Strategies

Susan Birne-Stone

Adrienne Cypres

Steven Winderbaum

Case management as a popular quality review strategy is a relatively recent phenomenon in behavioral health care. Historically, external reviews began at the hospital level in the mid-1970s (Goodman et al., 1992). At that time, written requests for more information were made after the patient completed inpatient psychiatric or chemical dependency treatment, or there was a retrospective review of the medical record. By the mid-1980s preauthorizations and concurrent reviews were being conducted for inpatient as well as outpatient care. This type of clinical case management was being applied to both hospital care and the work of private practitioners in an outpatient setting.

Today, there are many types of managed care organizations and benefit plans, such as the health maintenance organization (HMO), the preferred provider organization (PPO), and the point of service (POS) plan. Differences include the involvement of the primary care phycisian (PCP), internal versus external case management, and benefit reimbursement structures. Behavioral health care benefits are usually distinguished from other medical benefits and managed separately. It is the behavioral health care management program that is the focus of this chapter.

The coordination and provision of medically necessary treatment is at the core of effective behavioral health care. Case management for insurance beneficiaries works toward the development of an individualized treatment plan that sets a course toward a desired outcome. Progress is demonstrated through the achievement of specific, concretely defined goals set forth in the treatment plan and monitored through the follow-up concurrent review(s). In order to provide optimal services of behavioral health care delivery systems it is helpful to become familiar with the "maze" of managed care, which includes various roles, processes, and related concepts.

In this chapter we explore the application and implementation of managed care from a case manager's perspective, within the framework of inpatient and outpatient psychiatric and substance abuse treatment.

GENERAL CONCEPTS

Working within the context of behavioral health care, the patient is the eligible recipient of benefits as defined in a health insurance contract. This contract provides for the payment of a specified allotment of benefit (money, sessions, or days) in accordance with nationally recognized standards and norms of practice (Phillips & Wilson, 1993). The patient's diagnosis and clinical picture must be carefully assessed in order to ensure a proper fit between level of care, intensity of service, and treatment type. There is an intrinsic relationship between the concepts of assessment, diagnosis, treatment planning, and timely discharge. The framework provided by case management in managed behavioral health care capitalizes on this relationship by keeping planning focused on identifying specific goals and desired outcomes. It can be applied to a variety of modalities including cognitive, behavioral, and medical. It is an efficient approach that meets many needs while keeping the focus of treatment on the best interests of the patient.

With medical necessity (which will be defined later in this chapter) established, the patient becomes eligible to receive the approved benefits indicated in his or her insurance contract. By using the provisions of the insurance contract as a framework for decision making, the provider or clinician is better able to individualize treatment and deliver the optimal level of care in the context of available resources.

The managed care organization is the body responsible for overseeing services. Acting as a consultant, the clinical case manager works with the provider to determine the most efficient treatment available while maintaining the highest quality of care. The case manager ensures that the patient's severity of illness is matched to the appropriate intensity of service(s) (Phillips & Wilson, 1993).

Case management requires careful assessment, goal planning, and ongoing evaluation. Each of these activities is essential to outcome. The treatment plan and subsequent concurrent review(s) are the crucial tools of managing the treatment process in this type of health care model of case management. The result is a complete plan that keeps the presenting problem the focus of treatment. In order to clarify the relationship between problems, diagnosis, goals, and objectives it is helpful to view the treatment plan as a flowchart. The first step is the identification of symptoms and problems. This leads to a diagnosis and then the determination of goals and measurable objectives.

Concurrent review(s) are the ongoing reevaluations of this process until treatment is completed. An assessment should identify the patient's problems, strengths and weaknesses, and treatment or service needs. This provides the basis for diagnosis and for the determination of goals and objectives (Phillips & Wilson, 1993). A systematic collection of information gathered in accordance with the parameters set by the fourth edition of the *Diagnostic and Statistical Manual of Mental Disorders* or DSM-IV (A.P.A., 1994) and health care policy guidelines will support decisions made when determining goals. While assessment is comprehensive, it must also be clear and succinct. Identification of the most significant risk elements is crucial.

Interaction between significant areas of family functioning are noted. Significant problems caused, maintained or associated with identified dysfunctional behaviors are assessed by the practitioner and communicated to the clinical case manager.

Close consideration is given to major problem areas as reflected in a patient's level of functioning (Global Assessment of Functioning, A.P.A., 1994). The assessment of problems identifies what behavior or conditions need to be addressed. Related short- and long-term goals are established. By taking a small portion of a large problem and addressing it in an incremental manner, we increase the likelihood of verifiable progress.

With the problems and diagnosis clearly identified, a treatment plan is determined. Goals are framed and stated in order to address the behaviors and conditions raised in the assessment. The specific elements of the problem may be restated in terms of behavior or affect that needs to be diminished, alleviated, or abated.

With goals stated, objectives are determined. Objectives document the accomplishments that the patient will have made while achieving goals. They may be highly specific concrete tasks, demonstrated modifications in behavior, or other specific improvements in functioning. Objectives may be conceptualized as statements that will clearly indicate which behavior(s) will demonstrate that a patient's problem or condition has been addressed, reduced, or resolved. They state what can be expected to happen and can be used to measure progress and success.

Authorization

One of the most definitive elements of managed health care is the presence of an authorization system that serves multiple functions. It allows the case to be reviewed for medical necessity and offers the opportunity to channel care to the most appropriate form of treatment. There are several ways to obtain authorization, the most effective being a telephone-based system. This type of system relies on the subscriber, provider, or facility to call a central number and give information over the telephone. The advantage of this telephone-based system is the ability to be responsive in a timely manner. Specific procedures vary among different managed care companies.

Case Manager

Usually the clinical case manager—a licensed psychologist, social worker, or nurse—is the person responsible for the "management" of the patient's treatment episode. Important aspects of the clinical case manager's functions include assessment, referral, and coordination of care. The case manager is at the point of interface between the provider/facility and the managed care company.

It is with the case manager that the certification process begins, often with a call generated from a variety of sources including the client, a family member, a mental health professional, a physician, or a facility. The procedure that follows will be dependent on the type of call. When a subscriber or family member calls, it is usually for a referral, and the call is often precipitated by a crisis. Before making any type of referral, it is essential to make an assessment. The more precise the information the case manager has, the better he or she is able to determine appropriate treatment. Sometimes the beneficiary is unable to provide the necessary information due to intoxication or a psychiatric limitation, and a family member must be called upon. Often the caller has concerns about issues of confidentiality, particular whether his or her employer will have access to this information or will be notified about the call. Assurance of confidentiality is offered to allay such concerns. Often there is denial and/or a sense of shame on the part of the caller. It is important that the case manager keep this in mind and handle the situation with sensitivity.

Concurrent Review

Concurrent review occurs at intervals during the treatment process and allows for outcome assessment of patient progress and effectiveness of treatment. This process provides the opportunity to keep track of expected outcomes at certain predetermined points during an episode while keeping treatment focused. An episode of care is defined here as the length of treatment for a particular problem. Although new information and/or insights should be examined in the concurrent review, it is likely that more attention will be directed toward significant progress occurring since the initial assessment or last concurrent review. This type of review encourages a focus on the reduction of symptoms. It provides the opportunity to assess which interventions have been particularly successful or unsuccessful. Level of patient participation and willingness can be evaluated. A chance to update or revise diagnosis is given. The review(s) address any change in the patient's clinical status. Medical necessity is also reevaluated.

APPLICATION TO OUTPATIENT TREATMENT

Managed care clinicians are charged with the task of ensuring that subscribers receive medically necessary treatment at the most cost-effective level of care. To accomplish this for outpatient treatment, managed care companies have developed clinical policies and procedures on which decisions are based. Although specific policies vary, most managed care companies address the following questions:

- Is treatment medically necessary?
- Is the treatment plan consistent with national standards and guidelines for the diagnosis?
- Is the treatment plan time- and cost-sensitive?

Medical Necessity

In order to determine medical necessity, there first needs to be an assessment of the patient's presenting problem(s) with a focus on the current level of functioning. Treatment intended solely for self-improvement or for normal life stress reactions is not considered medically necessary. Most companies require the presence of a mental disorder as defined in DSM IV (1994), and will consider only an Axis I diagnosis as medically necessary. Treatment exclusively for an Axis II diagnosis is generally not reimbursed. Some companies do their own assessment with the patient either in person or on the telephone. Other companies rely on contracted providers to do the initial assessment. (It is important to know the specific policies of the managed care company under which the patient is covered.)

Most companies require a biopsychosocial assessment of the patient.

Such an assessment must include information about psychological, medical, family, vocational, and social factors. Substance dependence/abuse should be addressed as well as prior treatment history. The assessment must also include a full mental status examination as well as a statement of risk factors. In *Managing Managed Care*, Goodman and colleagues (1992) use the term *impairment* to describe the ". . . reasons why a patient requires treatment. They are not the reason(s) for the presence of the disorder, nor are they the disorder itself. Rather, they are observable, objectifiable manifestations that necessitate and justify care" (p. 31). They are the symptoms that need to be alleviated to enable the person to function at a reasonable level. When a case is being presented to a managed care clinician, the patient's impairment(s) must be defined, as they become the focus of treatment.

Treatment

Before the case manager authorizes reimbursement for treatment, medical necessity needs to be established. In addition to considering the patient's current level of functioning, there must be a reasonable expectation that the patient's condition will improve with treatment. In thinking about treatment, the view shared by most managed care practitioners is that the least invasive therapeutic intervention should be employed whenever possible. Since the most helpful treatment occurs in the most natural setting, outpatient care is usually preferable (Winegarin, 1992). Hospital-based treatment is usually reserved for patients who are too acutely ill to be treated on an outpatient basis. At the end of the assessment, a treatment intervention will be made, and if the clinical case manager thinks that inpatient hospitalization is appropriate, a particular facility, or several facilities, will be suggested.

Treatment plans must be consistent with the clinical picture presented in the assessment. Goals should be clear, measurable, and realistic; they should address the presenting problem. The focus should be on the alleviation of the patient's impairment(s) and increasing the level of functioning. Recommendations are expected to be consistent with national guidelines for the diagnosis (Phillips & Wilson, 1993). Consultations should be used when indicated—for example, medication evaluations, an area that is too often overlooked by social workers and psychologists. Many managed care clinicians find themselves recommending a medication evaluation where it has not been considered by the treating clinician. In such instances, medication has in fact been indicated and proven to be extremely effective. The most common symptoms that tend to be overlooked for medication evaluation are depression, anxiety, and panic attacks.

If a patient is receiving treatment by more than one provider, it is required that the primary therapist coordinate the treatment and have ongoing communication with all providers. Knowledge of dosage and frequency of medication is expected of the primary therapist. Use of community resources such as support groups should also be considered in formulating the discharge plan.

Time/Cost Factors

It is imperative that mental health providers give consideration to time and cost when planning treatment. If a patient's symptoms can be alleviated with brief focused treatment in 10 sessions, longer-term treatment will not be authorized for reimbursement. As we have mentioned, medication should also be considered for certain disorders.

Considerations for the Treatment of Children

Most managed care companies view child pathology within a biopsychosocial framework. Strong consideration is given to family issues in the assessment as well as in the treatment. Parents must be seen and included in the treatment. A family therapy model of treatment is usually preferred as the treatment of choice when indicated. Consultations may be required to make a differential diagnosis or for a medication evaluation. Psychological and neuropsychological testing must meet criteria for medical necessity; it is not conducted routinely. Reimbursement for a full battery of tests will not be given unless each test is clinically indicated. For example, psychological testing is not routinely needed to diagnose Attention Deficit Disorder (A.P.A., 1994). Psychological testing for educational purposes will usually not be reimbursed. It is expected that those tests will be conducted in the schools.

It is also expected that the treating clinician will rule out any type of maltreatment. If abuse or neglect is suspected, the clinician is required to contact Child Protective Services. Clinicians need to be particularly careful to explore substance abuse issues when working with adolescents, as this problem is often overlooked or minimized. It is important to coordinate services with the school when working with adolescents.

In order to help illustrate these concepts, the following case example is provided.

Mr. Williams called a managed care company inquiring about treatment for his 8-year-old son, John. He was referred to a clinical case manager, Ms. Smith, for an assessment. Mr. Williams said that John had been giving him a hard time. For the past three months John had been hyperactive, was not following rules, and was having difficulty concentrating on his homework. John was having difficulty in school, and his teacher complained that he had been disrupting the class. Mr. Williams had seen a television special on Attention Deficit Disorder (ADD) and was concerned that his son seemed to fit the profile.

The case manager asked Mr. Williams if he was aware of anything that happened three months ago, since that was when he reported the problems began. Mr. Williams explained that nothing happened at that time, but that six months ago he and his wife separated. He thought, however, that this was a good thing, since there was so much fighting when she was living with them. Mr. Williams did not believe that this was the source of his son's problems, since his 11-year-old daughter was doing great and she was trying to help John. Ms. Smith asked if John seemed sad or depressed, if he had temper tantrums or was violent. Mr. Williams said he seemed angry, stamping his feet, and one time threw something at his sister, but it missed her. He also reported, when asked, that John does wake up in the middle of the night and says he has bad dreams but won't talk about them. Mr. Williams reported no medical problems or prior treatment, although he said his wife needed treatment. Ms. Smith inquired about John's contact with his mother. Mrs. Williams was supposed to see John on the weekends, although she regularly failed to follow through. Ms. Smith explained that it seemed to have been a difficult year for everyone and referred John to Ms. Ray, a social worker who specializes in family treatment of children and adolescents. The case manager authorized five sessions for assessment and told Mr. Williams to have the therapist call her after the family had been seen. Ms. Smith also would be calling Ms. Ray to inform her of the referral.

Ms. Smith contacted Ms. Ray and discussed the case. Then, after having individual sessions with the father, son, and mother, and a family session with the father and two children, Ms. Ray called Ms. Smith. Ms. Ray also had phone contact with John's teacher and guidance counselor. Ms. Ray reported that it appeared that John was in fact reacting to the parent's separation and disappointments regarding his mother's failed visits. There was not at that time evidence that John had ADD. John was very verbal during sessions and was able to express his anger at his sister for trying to be his mother as well as his sadness regarding his mother.

A treatment plan was developed with the family that included the following goals: John would improve—in school, his homework, his relationship with his dad and sister—and he would express his negative feelings in more constructive ways. Other goals were related to Mr. and Mrs. William's parenting techniques, since they had agreed to have a session to discuss the children. Ms. Ray was also going to work with the school and John was going to see the guidance counselor to work on school problems.

A total of 10 individual sessions and 10 family sessions were authorized over a 6-month period. At the end of the authorization period, Ms. Ray called and said that John was doing better. Most of the goals had been met. Eight individual sessions and six family sessions had been used. The total number, including the original assessment, was 18 sessions. Treatment was terminated and Mr. Williams was referred to a parents' support group in his local church. Mr. and Mrs. Williams were also referred to a divorce mediator to help them with their divorce. Both John and his sister were referred to an after-school program and were receiving counseling in their schools. Ms. Ray would contact the family in 3 months for a follow-up, and they knew they could call on her if needed.

APPLICATION TO INPATIENT TREATMENT

As inpatient care is the most expensive component of a managed health care system, it requires the most intense level of case management. Since timeliness is such an important factor in managing inpatient cases, it is essential that the hospital or facility notify the managed care company within 48 hours of the admission and that the case manager do an initial evaluation as quickly as possible, with either the attending psychiatrist, psychotherapist, or a utilization review nurse. The assessment process will focus on presenting symptoms, history of psychiatric or substance abuse, other medical conditions, DSM-IV (1994) diagnosis on all five axes, and any other information that seems relevant to the clinical picture. Treatment will be discussed, as will tentative discharge plans and discharge date. If the patient meets the criteria for medical necessity and the treatment proposed seems appropriate, the case manager will authorize the treatment and approve between one and five days. At the end of that time the case manager will contact the provider again and get a clinical update—that is, a concurrent review. If the patient seems improved but not yet returned to a baseline or normal level of functioning and still meets criteria for medical necessity, the treatment plan will be discussed; if appropriate, more days can be approved. If the patient is not showing any signs of expected improvement, the treatment plan needs to be reevaluated. Again, more days could be authorized, but the case manager must always be mindful of the length of stay and ensure that these days are used optimally, since treatment in many hospitals is benefit-driven. The case manager must be aware of the medication the patient is receiving and check that it is appropriate for the patient's diagnosis. Doses must be at therapeutic levels; when they are not, it is important to understand why in order to clarify the treatment rationale.

The two categories of cases that are referred to a case manager for inpatient assessment are psychiatric and substance abuse. The psychiatric cases are typically for depression, suicidal or homicidal ideation, bipolar disorder, and an exacerbation of a psychotic disorder. Admissions are for Axis I diagnoses only (A.P.A., 1994). The focus of treatment is on the acute episode, with the aim of stabilizing patients and returning them to their previous level of functioning.

A large percentage of the patients referred to a case manager for assessment are seeking treatment for substance abuse. Substance abuse treatment can be broken down into two different types or categories, detoxification and rehabilitation. Detoxification is the medical treatment for alcohol or substance dependence or withdrawal. Traditionally this has been done in an inpatient facility, though more recently outpatient programs have been developed. Concurrent mental illness is evaluated and treated as a part of the process. Referrals for ongoing rehabilitation services are made as needed.

A rehabilitation program provides multiple intensive nonresidential services to patients diagnosed as substance abusers or substance dependent. Treatment is done by a multidisciplinary staff under the direction of a qualified health professional. Programs are either full- or part-time and involve treatment on a daily basis (N.Y. State Department of Social Services, 1992).

The following case examples are common clinical presentations and are used to illustrate the assessment process in substance abuse cases.

Case #1

Tom is a 44-year-old single employed male. He called the managed care company asking for approval to a specific substance abuse facility, one that is very popular due to its frequent television advertising. He wanted to go into an alcohol rehabilitation program for his drinking problem. He told the case manager that he was depressed and that this made him drink. Several months earlier he had been in a psychiatric hospital, but he said that he was duped into a voluntary admission, believing that he was going to get treatment for his alcohol problem. Somehow, the doctor who admitted him thought he was a suicide risk. Tom denied suicidal ideation but did say that he was feeling hopeless. He signed himself out of that hospital after 3 days. But last month, after a drinking binge, was picked up by the police and brought to the emergency room of a large city hospital. He was also admitted to that hospital's psychiatric unit and released in a few days. Tom denies any psychiatric history, reiterating that his problem is the alcohol. He is a binge drinker who is unable to stop once he starts. He has been drinking for about 5 years and has occasional blackouts but no seizures. Significant medical history or current medical problems were denied. He denies D.W.I.'s or other legal problems. He also denies prior substance abuse treatment; has never had an alcohol detoxification but has been to AA meetings once or twice.

Case #2

Jim is a 55-year-old married retired male. He also called the managed care company asking for approval of a detoxification for his alcohol problem. He had been drinking for more than 25 years and had been through a detoxification approximately 10 years earlier. He had never been in a rehabilitation program. He drinks about a half gallon of wine daily and sometimes additional beer. He denied any other substance abuse, suicidal or homicidal ideation, and had no known psychiatric history. He was given approval for a detox. When he arrived at the hospital, he suffered a seizure in the admitting office. The nurse then called the managed care company to advise them of the situation. She thought that he might be having a stroke and stated that he was currently on a medical unit. After a week, the hospital called the managed care company and reported that the patient was stable but that he had high blood pressure and elevated liver enzymes. They requested that he be transferred to a substance abuse rehab unit.

How does the case manager determine the appropriate level of treatment for these two people? Although these two cases appear to be similar, the recommendations for treatment are quite different. Each patient has a problem with alcohol but neither one is abusing any other substance. Nor does either one have any prior psychiatric history. Do they each need the same level of care?

In our case examples, Jim (Case #2) was approved for inpatient treatment because of his medical problems, which were considered to be potentially life-threatening. Tom (Case #1) was referred to detox, to be followed by intensive outpatient treatment in a dual diagnosis program because of his depression. It has been estimated that up to 30% of chemically dependent patients also have an additional mental disorder (Miller et al., 1986). Sometimes a psychiatric disorder precedes the substance abuse and may have a role in its development. In these cases the psychiatric disorder and the addiction make up the primary diagnosis. Secondary addictions are usually considered to be more difficult to treat (Austed & Berman, 1991). From 10 to 15% of chemically addicted patients have diagnosable affective disorders, and 7 to 10% have anxiety and panic disorders (Austed & Berman).

An assessment that includes as much of this information as possible will help to determine the appropriate level of care. A detox may be necessary if the person has been using alcohol or other physically addictive substances. Detox from heroin is common because of the discomfort of the withdrawal, but cocaine does not require a detox. In some cases the detox can be used as a springboard for further inpatient treatment and in other cases for outpatient treatment. Although most companies have criteria to determine levels of treatment, the recommendation is usually determined on a case-by-case basis. Contrary to popular myth, there is no empiric evidence to suggest that inpatient rehab leads to more successful outcomes than outpatient rehab.

Research in the area of substance abuse treatment has not shown that fixed-length treatment provides superior results as compared with outpatient care (Miller, Williams, & Reid, 1986). In their review, Miller et al. (1986) found that controlled comparisons consistently demonstrated no overall advantage for inpatient over outpatient treatment, for longer over shorter inpatient programs, or for more intensive over less intensive intervention in the treatment of substance abuse. Increasingly, inpatient care is used primarily for detox or for short periods of treatment when the patient has medical complications or lives with a substance-abusing spouse. While decisions are made on a case-by-case basis, inpatient treatment is not usually approved unless the patient has failed at outpatient treatment in the past.

Inpatient treatment is not usually the first line of treatment and is usually not recommended for someone who has had no past outpatient treatment.

It may be recommended for someone who has a long history of substance abuse and has had previous treatment and had really made the attempt to stop or for someone who has had a long period of recovery and is in a program but had a relapse.

The following factors need to be addressed in making the substance abuse assessment:

1. *Presenting problem.* What is the person currently using, how much and how often, and when did he or she begin? A medical assessment prior to treatment is essential, as abrupt withdrawal from alcohol and certain medications can result in seizures or strokes.
2. *Medical history.* Both present and past.
3. *Psychiatric history, both present and past.* Is the person currently being treated? If so how? Where? By whom? List any past treatment.
4. *Treatment history.* Has the person ever been treated for this problem before? When? Where? If this is a relapse, when did it occur? What were the stressors around that time? Length of time of recovery.
5. *Level of functioning.* Does the person work and is he or she able to work currently? Is the person's job in jeopardy? How long has the person been working and what kind of work does he or she do? Does the person have a family? Does their spouse or partner use? Is there any support system?

Some Considerations for Substance Abuse Problems

If a patient is actively abusing any substance, in- or outpatient mental health treatment will not be authorized for reimbursement. The first goal with a substance abuser is abstinence. Most managed care companies will authorize substance abuse treatment only with licensed facilities as opposed to private individuals or groups. Use of 12-step programs is strongly recommended.

Discharge Planning

Discharge planning is a very important part of the treatment process. Patients discharged from psychiatric hospitals are often at high risk, so it is essential that they have an aftercare appointment scheduled within a short time of the discharge. Partial day-hospital programs can prevent a hospitalization or act as a bridge after discharge. It can help the patient make a successful transition back into the community. Such programs are designed for patients with serious disorders that require more intensive and comprehensive treatment than can be provided in an outpatient setting. However, not all policies have this option; even when they do, it is often part of the inpatient hospital benefit. Sometimes those days can be authorized by substituting benefits in a ratio of outpatient to inpatient days. While partial hospitalization can be very helpful for many patients, substituting benefits has potential pitfalls. If patients use up their inpatient benefits and then require more hospitalization, they will often have to pay for this treatment themselves. However, if it will shorten the hospital stay or keep the patient from needing to be readmitted, such a risk may be worth taking.

Emergency Intervention

An essential aspect of managed mental health care is emergency intervention. Crises occur at all hours, so there must be a system in place to deal with them. Prompt intervention can result in a diversion to outpatient treatment instead of costly hospitalization. When a call comes in after regular business hours, it is often relayed to an answering service or a paging system. In most companies, clinical case managers are on call and available to handle these emergency situations. Their assessment will focus on the presenting symptoms and on potential for risk. Often an overnight in the hospital will be authorized if it seems to meet the criteria of medical necessity; this judgment will be made primarily on the basis of the presenting symptoms. The case will then be reviewed during regular business hours by the assigned case manager.

Denials

Often patients are admitted to the hospital without preauthorization. Sometimes it is an emergency admission, but often the hospital does not notify the managed care company for 48 hours or more. If the lapse is more than 72 hours, authorization payment will not be given and the facility will be advised that they have had an administrative denial of payment for services. This will be followed up with a letter explaining the reason for the denial and the procedure for an appeal. Appeal is an option always open to every provider and facility. They are asked to explain in writing why they did not comply with the managed care guidelines for notification of admission. The appeal will be presented to a committee, who will decide on the merits of the explanation. If the denial is upheld, the facility will be notified of this in writing. If the denial is overturned, medical records will be requested and an assessment of the medical necessity for the treatment will be done retrospectively.

Particular attention will be paid to the presenting problem, as well as the history, diagnosis, medications, and treatment plans. Length of stay and discharge plans will also be noted. The case manager will be evaluating the treatment in terms of clinical picture; e.g., do the medications and doses fit the diagnosis and the severity of illness? Did this patient receive some kind of therapy? If so, what kind? Is the psychiatrist seeing this patient daily? If it is determined that the treatment is both medically necessary and appropriate, an approval will be given and the hospital will be reimbursed by the patient's company. If the case manager determines that the treatment is either not medically necessary, not appropriate, or both, he or she will consult with one of the managed care psychiatrists. If it is determined that the treatment was not necessary and/or appropriate, the facility will be advised of a denial of payment and they will not be reimbursed by the patient's third-party payor.

CONCLUSION

This chapter has examined the growing use of case management as a quality review strategy in behavioral health care. Key concepts and core principles have been defined and related to both inpatient and outpatient treatment. We have seen how the traditional health care practices of assessment, treatment planning, and discharge planning are capitalized on in managed care and used as tools to promote efficiency and effectiveness. We have also seen how a diagnosis of mental illness and the assessment of patient level of functioning can be translated into the determination of observable goals. The achievement of these goals, as reflected by changes in the GAF score, provides us with concrete markers that indicate progress.

The roles and functions of the case manager and the treatment provider have been defined as well. The role of the provider remains unchanged. Through the use of the patient/therapist relationship, he or she provides treatment in accordance with his or her discipline, training, and experience. The clinical case manager is the person responsible for the management of the patient's benefit. The clinical case manager works with the provider to ensure maximum use of the patient's available health care benefits in accordance with the parameters set forth by the individual insurance policy. Management decisions are based on the assessment determined in conjunction with the provider. The clinical case manager assures a proper fit between level of required care, intensity of service, and type of treatment.

As the millennium approaches, we find the behavioral health care industry undergoing significant changes. Core theories of psychotherapy remain in place, but new approaches abound. There is a call to deliver adequate health care fairly to all. While treatment is always considered on a case-by-case basis, a certain level of consistency with regard to prognosis must be offered. The realities of life in a changing industry and society present the clinician with new challenges. The framework provided by case management in managed care addresses these challenges in a realistic and adaptable manner.

REFERENCES

A.P.A. (1994). *Diagnostic statistical manual of mental disorders* (DSM-IV). Washington, DC: American Psychiatric Association.

Austed, C., & Berman, W. H. (1991). *Psychotherapy in managed care: The optimal use of time and resources*. Washington, DC: American Psychological Association.

Endicott, J., Spitzer, R., Fliess, J., & Cohen, J. (1975). *The Global Assessment Scale.* New York: New York Department of Mental Hygiene.

Feldman, S. (1992). *Managed Mental Health Services.* Springfield, IL: Charles C Thomas.

Goodman, M., Brown, J., & Deitz, P. (1992). *Managing managed care.* Washington, DC: American Psychiatric Press.

Miller, K. Williams, R., & Reid, K. (1986). Inpatient alcoholism treatment: Who benefits? *American Psychologist, 41,* 794–805.

N.Y. State Department of Social Services (1993). *Comprehensive Plan and Update for Alcohol and Substance Abuse Services in New York State.* (1992), 27–29.

Phillips, K., & Wilson, G. (1993). Concepts and definitions used in quality assurance and utilization review, in *Manual of psychiatric quality assurance.* Washington, DC: American Psychiatric Association.

Winegarin, N. (1992). *The clinician's guide to managed health care.* Binghamton, NY: Haworth Press.

CHAPTER 4

When to Consider a Psychopharmacologic Intervention

Kelley L. Phillips

How does one figure out the right moment to involve a specialist in enhancing a treatment so that the patient is able to recover better and faster? Specifically, when does one refer a patient for a medication consult? Equally important, how do you know that the consultant you have chosen is competent and reliable for the patient you refer?

It is difficult to be an effective therapist today, with the increased expectations to provide optimal impact on patient outcome, without establishing some linkage with a multidisciplinary team. How does one shift from being a solo practitioner of psychotherapy to becoming a member of a health care team, so that excellent, coordinated, integrated services are provided for your patient population (Donabedian, 1980)? A useful strategy is to develop relationships with clinicians who are involved in a quality managed care network or linked electronically with ongoing updates of clinical decision guidelines and patient outcomes, so that you are assured that your health care team is providing state-of-the-art services and consultation (Eddy, 1990; Fawcett, 1994).

The technology age has brought us new ways of learning as well as a demand for an increased pace in our knowledge base for delivery of clinical services. This means considering a different methodology in learning, since

---

Note: See the Appendix at the end of this chapter (p. 73) for definitions of words that appear in *italics*.

our old ways are too slow and unreliable. We need to be checking out the technology and clinical guideline topics at professional meetings as well as interviewing those people who participate in these presentations and using our computers as our key teaching aids to link up electronically with clinical bulletin boards (Miller, 1994; Brown-Beasley, 1994; Lieff, 1994).

The first professional liaison nonmedical psychotherapists should consider developing is with psychiatrists, since severity of illness—for example, severe depression and/or suicidality or psychosis—is the most important issue requiring consultation in a psychotherapy practice. If such a practice includes a large population of patients with a particular diagnosis (such as attention deficit, eating disorder, or chemical dependence), it is useful to find a match with one or more psychiatrists who also have that particular population and expertise in their practices.

For those psychotherapists who have individual practices, it is key to meet with prospective referral sources. Too often, we know about clinicians only by word of mouth and are not able to be specific about their practices and treatment styles. Check out the following:

- Their philosophy of care
- Their expertise in psychopharmacology
- Their treatment strategies about gender differences
- Whether they currently provide inpatient care and what percentage of their practice this represents
- How they handle referrals

Philosophy of care is relevant. Is this psychiatrist committed to working with patients using a health model rather than an illness model? An important part of this model is integrated care, with the patient as a partner in the plan.

It is significant to hear that a general psychiatrist takes a nationally recognized annual psychopharmacology update course or is on the "internet" to access specialist consultations. To match the description of a psychopharmacology specialist or subspecialist, a psychiatrist must have relevant formal psychopharmacology training in addition to training in general psychiatry, such as three years of clinical research at the National Institutes of Health.

There are significant gender differences to consider when using medications, such as dose amount, variance in drug uptake and metabolism across the menstrual and life cycle, and side-effects profile. For those psychiatrists selected for your patient referral who trained prior to the 1980s, when gender issues started having an impact on research design, it is important to clarify how and whether the consultant has kept up with this new information about gender. You might ask how the psychiatrist evaluates and treats medication response in women throughout the menstrual cycle. Or you might ask for specific examples of patients the psychiatrist has treated in his or her own practice—both those that were successful and those that were not so successful.

It is important to know whether the consultant psychiatrist maintains a hospital practice and, if not, what his or her process is for hospitalizing patients. Patients are not optimally taken care of if the psychiatrist follows only a couple of hospitalized patients a year. This is the same concept as being required to deliver a certain number of babies a year to maintain those skill sets and privileges. A multidisciplinary team concept with dedicated hospital physician staff for a group of hospitalized patients is a more coordinated approach with better patient outcomes.

Assessment tools (see Exhibit 4.1), both paper-based and electronically recorded, have greatly assisted in quantifying and communicating patient changes in mood and behavior. It is useful to explore which tools the consultant psychiatrist uses in patient care and how he or she shares this information with patients and their health care teams. It is important to incorporate some of these tools into your own practice. Also, it is relevant to see consultants' offices and to know their office hours and work patterns. This takes more time and effort; however, it has become a "gold standard" (Klein, 1994).

Referral sources are bidirectional. A psychiatrist is much more interested in referring to someone whom he or she has met—who has been specific in learning about the psychiatrist's practice and has educated the psychiatrist about his or her own areas of expertise and style of work—than to someone about whom less information is available.

Patient evaluation and referral skills need to meet quality standards. Nonphysician psychotherapists err far more on the side of omission than commission by not obtaining a more detailed and specific history about symptoms, family, chemical dependence, for example, leading to delay of an accurate diagnosis and appropriate treatment plan. This results in the waste of tremendous human and dollar resources. Physicians also waste tremendous resources, usually by commission errors of overutilization or mismatching of services.

We often fool ourselves into thinking that usual and customary practice is state-of-the-art or optimal practice when the reality is that it often has no scientific basis whatsoever. In another era, bloodletting was a usual and customary practice. The healers felt relieved that they were not beheaded, although patients sometimes died from their treatment. This practice was not based on science. Currently, we are often swayed by the full-court press of marketing—in an attempt to have a state-of-the-art practice—to believe that the most expensive or newest medication is best. In fact, it is often the most expensive but no more effective than the less expensive proven drugs.

FRAMEWORK FOR EVALUATION AND REFERRAL

A public health approach to patient care is selected as the model for early intervention, coordinated delivery of services, and improved outcomes in patients' health status.

A fundamental touchstone of this approach is an accurate, comprehensive, and timely assessment. It includes a *biopsychosocial* framework with an appropriately matched treatment plan as the starting point of each and every intervention. This frame includes performing a *mental status examination*; developing a comprehensive formulation and *differential diagnosis*; identifying the severity of illness with clinical rationale; evaluating the biological, family, and social context of the person; and then matching these findings with a treatment plan that will achieve an optimal patient outcome.

The mental status exam is conducted while the history and current status are elicited. A major component is observation. One observes whether the patient is disheveled or diaphoretic; what kind of gait he or she has; characteristic patient gestures; and whether there are any tics or restlessness. This assists in determining a decrease in energy for self-care, whether the patient is intoxicated or possibly in withdrawal, or whether he or she has a neurologic or endocrine illness. Speech, thought content, perception, affect, and cognition round out the exam.

When the patient assessment is falling into place, an individualized, matched plan of action is the next step. Key components of the treatment plan are identifying what problem(s) will be addressed, establishing in what and how the patient will make progress, and specifying the time frame in which this outcome will occur.

In an attempt to enhance the consistency and *reliability* of our clinical practices, a specific scientific clinical decision-making process called an *algorithm* has been developed. Also, as clinical findings are more rigorously evaluated, the *validity* of a particular approach is clarified.

Depression is selected as the most appropriate clinical problem to consider in using an algorithm, since it is such a pervasive illness and is the most frequent reason for patient referral for a psychiatric evaluation—see *secondary care* and *tertiary care* (Klein, 1994; Weissman, 1987). Depression presents itself in many forms—as a major depressive illness or as a form of bipolar illness; it combines with personality disorders, chemical dependence, and other medical and psychiatric conditions; it can also result from the use of certain medications. It has significant treatment variations based on gender—such as pregnancy, phase of menstrual cycle, and menopause—as well as on the age of the patient.

The algorithm in Exhibit 4.1 highlights the critical common pathway for clinical decision making, assessment, and time lines in the treatment of a problem of depression.

Formalized tools, such as self-report questionnaires or interactive ones involving therapist and patient assist the clinician in a timely fashion, quantifying the level of an individual's depression as well as helping to identify specific key individual characteristics that are important for treatment. Five frequently used tools are highlighted for ease of therapist selection.

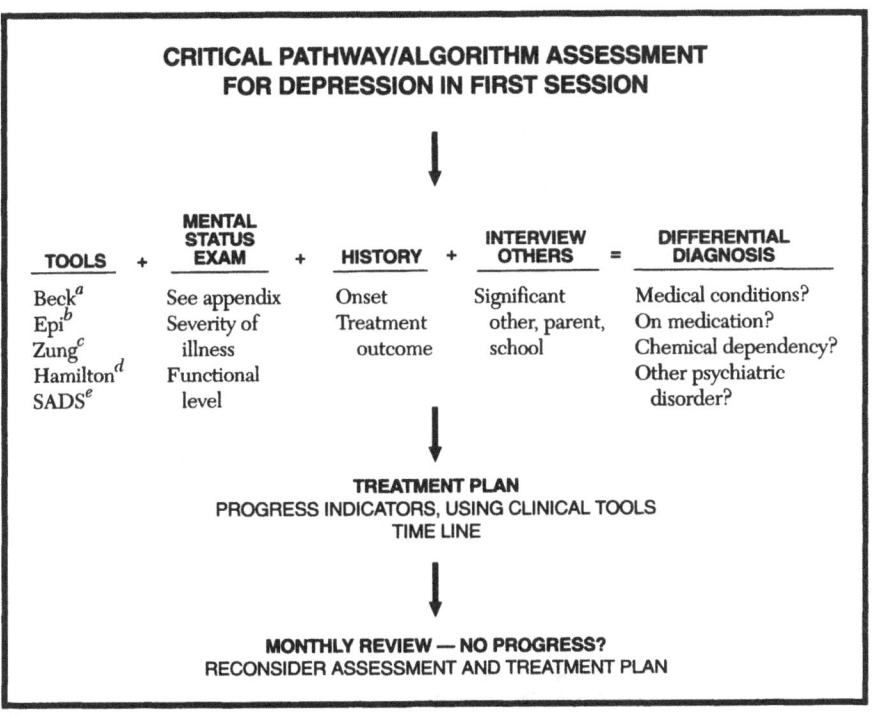

CRITICAL PATHWAY/ALGORITHM ASSESSMENT
FOR DEPRESSION IN FIRST SESSION

TOOLS +	MENTAL STATUS EXAM +	HISTORY +	INTERVIEW OTHERS =	DIFFERENTIAL DIAGNOSIS
Beck[a] Epi[b] Zung[c] Hamilton[d] SADS[e]	See appendix Severity of illness Functional level	Onset Treatment outcome	Significant other, parent, school	Medical conditions? On medication? Chemical dependency? Other psychiatric disorder?

TREATMENT PLAN
PROGRESS INDICATORS, USING CLINICAL TOOLS
TIME LINE

MONTHLY REVIEW — NO PROGRESS?
RECONSIDER ASSESSMENT AND TREATMENT PLAN

[a]Beck Depression Inventory
[b]Center for Epidemiological Studies — Depression (Radloff)
[c]Zung Self-Rating Depression Scale
[d]Hamilton Rating Scale
[e]Schedule for Affective Disorders + Schizophrenia (Endicott)

Exhibit 4.1. Assessment

The Beck Depression Inventory (BDI: Beck et al., 1961), the Center for Epidemiological Studies-Depression Scale (CES-D: Radloff, 1977), and the Zung self-rating depression scale (Zung, 1965) (see Exhibits 4.2A and 4.2B) are patient self-report questionnaires. Clinician rating scales include

---

PATIENT NAME

AGE _____ SEX _____ DATE _____

Please check a response for each of the 20 items.	None OR a Little of the Time	Some of the Time	Good Part of the Time	Most OR All of the Time
1. I FEEL DOWNHEARTED, BLUE, AND SAD	○	○	○	○
2. MORNING IS WHEN I FEEL THE BEST	○	○	○	○
3. I HAVE CRYING SPELLS OR FEEL LIKE IT	○	○	○	○
4. I HAVE TROUBLE SLEEPING THROUGH THE NIGHT	○	○	○	○
5. I EAT AS MUCH AS I USED TO	○	○	○	○
6. I ENJOY LOOKING AT, TALKING TO, AND BEING WITH ATTRACTIVE WOMEN/MEN	○	○	○	○
7. I NOTICE THAT I AM LOSING WEIGHT	○	○	○	○
8. I HAVE TROUBLE WITH CONSTIPATION	○	○	○	○
9. MY HEART BEATS FASTER THAN USUAL	○	○	○	○
10. I GET TIRED FOR NO REASON	○	○	○	○
11. MY MIND IS AS CLEAR AS IT USED TO BE	○	○	○	○
12. I FIND IT EASY TO DO THE THINGS I USED TO DO	○	○	○	○
13. I AM RESTLESS AND CAN'T KEEP STILL	○	○	○	○
14. I FEEL HOPEFUL ABOUT THE FUTURE	○	○	○	○
15. I AM MORE IRRITABLE THAN USUAL	○	○	○	○
16. I FIND IT EASY TO MAKE DECISIONS	○	○	○	○
17. I FEEL THAT I AM USEFUL AND NEEDED	○	○	○	○
18. MY LIFE IS PRETTY FULL	○	○	○	○
19. I FEEL THAT OTHERS WOULD BE BETTER OFF IF I WERE DEAD	○	○	○	○
20. I STILL ENJOY THE THINGS I USED TO DO	○	○	○	○

INSTRUCTIONS

Read each sentence carefully. For each statement, check the bubble in the column that best corresponds to how often you have felt that way during the past two weeks.

For statements 5 and 7, if you are on a diet, answer as if you were not.

Exhibit 4.2A. Zung Self-Rating Scale for Depression, Instructions.

PATIENT NAME _____

AGE _____ SEX _____ DATE _____

Please check a response for each of the 20 items.	None OR a Little of the Time	Some of the Time	Good Part of the Time	Most OR All of the Time
1. I FEEL DOWNHEARTED, BLUE, AND SAD	○ 1	○ 2	○ 3	○ 4
2. MORNING IS WHEN I FEEL THE BEST*	○ 4	○ 3	○ 2	○ 1
3. I HAVE CRYING SPELLS OR FEEL LIKE IT	○ 1	○ 2	○ 3	○ 4
4. I HAVE TROUBLE SLEEPING THROUGH THE NIGHT	○ 1	○ 2	○ 3	○ 4
5. I EAT AS MUCH AS I USED TO*	○ 4	○ 3	○ 2	○ 1
6. I ENJOY LOOKING AT, TALKING TO, AND BEING WITH ATTRACTIVE WOMEN/MEN*	○ 4	○ 3	○ 2	○ 1
7. I NOTICE THAT I AM LOSING WEIGHT	○ 1	○ 2	○ 3	○ 4
8. I HAVE TROUBLE WITH CONSTIPATION	○ 1	○ 2	○ 3	○ 4
9. MY HEART BEATS FASTER THAN USUAL	○ 1	○ 2	○ 3	○ 4
10. I GET TIRED FOR NO REASON	○ 1	○ 2	○ 3	○ 4
11. MY MIND IS AS CLEAR AS IT USED TO BE*	○ 4	○ 3	○ 2	○ 1
12. I FIND IT EASY TO DO THE THINGS I USED TO DO*	○ 4	○ 3	○ 2	○ 1
13. I AM RESTLESS AND CAN'T KEEP STILL	○ 1	○ 2	○ 3	○ 4
14. I FEEL HOPEFUL ABOUT THE FUTURE*	○ 4	○ 3	○ 2	○ 1
15. I AM MORE IRRITABLE THAN USUAL	○ 1	○ 2	○ 3	○ 4
16. I FIND IT EASY TO MAKE DECISIONS*	○ 4	○ 3	○ 2	○ 1
17. I FEEL THAT I AM USEFUL AND NEEDED*	○ 4	○ 3	○ 2	○ 1
18. MY LIFE IS PRETTY FULL*	○ 4	○ 3	○ 2	○ 1
19. I FEEL THAT OTHERS WOULD BE BETTER OFF IF I WERE DEAD	○ 1	○ 2	○ 3	○ 4
20. I STILL ENJOY THE THINGS I USED TO DO*	○ 4	○ 3	○ 2	○ 1

RAW SCORE

SDS INDEX

SDS Index*	Equivalent Clinical Global Impressions
Below-50	Within normal range, no psychopathology
50-59	Presence of minimal to mild depression
60-69	Presence of moderate to marked depression
70 and over	Presence of severe to extreme depression

Conversion of Raw Scores to the SDS Index

Raw Score	SDS Index	Raw Score	SDS Index	Raw Score	SDS Index	Raw Score	SDS Index	Raw Score	SDS Index
20	25	32	40	44	55	56	70	68	85
21	26	33	41	45	56	57	71	69	86
22	28	34	43	46	58	58	73	70	88
23	29	35	44	47	59	59	74	71	89
24	30	36	45	48	60	60	75	72	90
25	31	37	46	49	61	61	76	73	91
26	33	38	48	50	63	62	78	74	92
27	34	39	49	51	64	63	79	75	94
28	35	40	50	52	65	64	80	76	95
29	36	41	51	53	66	65	81	77	96
30	38	42	53	54	68	66	83	78	98
31	39	43	54	55	69	67	84	79	99
								80	100

*Severity of depression score

Exhibit 4.2B. Zung Self-Rating Scale for Depression, Scoring Form.

the Hamilton Rating Scale for Depression (HRS-D: Hamilton, 1960) and the Schedule for Affective Disorders and Schizophrenia (SADS: Endicott et al., 1978). Scores over 20 on the Beck or the Hamilton, over 60 on the Zung, or over 40 on the CES-D suggest that a patient is experiencing sufficient severity of depression that referral for a psychopharmacologic assessment be considered.

Key elements to be clarified in evaluating a patient's mental status are suicide ideation, plan, lethality, intention and access to means of performing the act; amount of sleep and appetite disturbance; disturbance in concentration and ability to maintain cognitive functioning; and mood disturbance and ability to enjoy life. Onset of change in mood, personal and family history of depression, physical illness, chemical dependence, as well as medication history are relevant parts for the assessment. The patient's history of impulsive behavior and outcomes as well as her or his social support system are critical data to incorporate for planning the most appropriate treatment intervention.

Suicidality is an essential subject to explore. Some patients think about suicide but state that they could not commit the act for religious reasons, because of parental responsibilities, or for fear of doing psychic harm to loved ones. It is important to find out how frequently these thoughts occur and what the patient does to get rid of them—and whether the patient worries that he or she will not be able to control such actions. The more impulsive one is and the more intrusive these thoughts are, the greater the risk of taking some action. Others have a plan of action including time, place, and weapon. It is critical to learn about this plan in detail, access to weapon, and whether it involves hurting others. Some people are delusional, grandiose, or under the influence of drugs or alcohol; thus, with their judgment impaired, they are at higher risk of injuring themselves. Some are worried that they will not be able to resist their impulses to drive off the road.

A patient's appearance and gait are the first components a clinician assesses to integrate into his or her evaluation. Grooming, posture, dress, mannerisms, and gestures all contribute to an understanding how well patients are feeling about themselves and how much energy they have to respond to personal, ethnic, and cultural expectations. Some knowledge about one's patients' spirituality and religious beliefs is also essential to an understanding of their normal ways of experiencing their world.

A family member, significant other, teacher, parent, or child is a key asset in assisting with a fuller description of a patient's current functional status as well as helping with the identification of recent changes in that status. For adult patients, a work history is very informative for ascertaining work role level of functioning. How one cares for one's children is very telling about how creative a parent is in using resources, skills, and abilities. All this clinical information is integrated in the development of a differential diagnosis using these tools, and in information gathering to enhance one's clinical acumen. This process includes a primary diagnosis—which is a working diagnosis—and which is justified by one's clinical rationale. Rule-out diagnoses identify those clinical problems which, with more clinical information, are added to the primary diagnosis and will impact the patient's treatment plan, or are excluded.

It is relevant to sort out the severity of the individual's problem and the change in severity over the previous year by using the Global Assessment of Functioning scale (GAF), which is Axis V of the fourth edition of the *Diagnostic and Statistical Manual of Mental Disorders* (American Psychiatric Association, 1994). Many therapists are not very experienced and do not use this scale accurately. It is useful to refine these skills, since it will enable one to better and more accurately communicate what is happening with one's patient. Description and references of GAF are found in the section titled "Multiaxial Assessment" in DSM-IV, pages 25 through 35 (A.P.A., 1994).

Tremendous amounts of new knowledge and information need to be incorporated into our work, which has become much more detailed and refined. A completed assessment, for example, is usually accomplished in one session; it sometimes needs two and rarely requires three sessions.

Evaluating a patient's progress is another important consideration in patient care. A general guideline as to when to consider a consultation in an outpatient setting is if the patient's progress is not timely—that is, if there is no progress in a month. Then, perhaps more than one or a different treatment intervention needs to be considered. Patient dropout rate is high if there is no relief/support in this time period (see Exhibit 4.1). A patient self-rating scale is often useful to follow his or her progress (see Exhibit 4.2B).

TEAMWORK

Many clinicians find that their patients refuse medications. There is a body of scientific literature demonstrating that medications are an effective and essential treatment component for most psychiatric and chemical dependency illnesses. Examples include major depression, bipolar illness, schizophrenia, alcohol and opioid dependence, attention deficit hyperactivity disorder, and many personality disorders (DSM-IV, Axis II) (Karusu, 1989).

If a person's problem can be resolved faster with a combined treatment intervention of a particular psychotherapy and medication than with a single strategy, this is considered the *optimal* treatment approach and is derived using a *cost/benefit* perspective. It is in the best interest of patients for all clinicians to offer an optimal treatment plan. If the patient and therapist are not in harmony with the proposed treatment plan, then it is difficult for either party to perform well. A second opinion, referral for a medication consultation, or referral to another therapist are all good strategies for excellent care. If a patient refuses these, consult with a colleague experienced in these issues and with your malpractice organization. A letter to as well as telephone contact with the patient identifying a particular expert who is willing to continue work with the patient is in order and usually ends your responsibility. If the patient is dangerous, that is, suicidal or homicidal, it is obligatory to attempt to have the patient examined and possibly committed to a safer environment. This is where your team and electronic bulletin board can be critical in maintaining your edge.

If your patient refuses your proposed plan, then you, as a skilled clinician, do not stay involved in providing less than optimal care. In this situation, precious resources are being utilized poorly, and the public is not willing to pay for inefficiencies and suboptimal care.

Giving patients reading materials to learn more about their illness and treatment options often assist them in choosing a good treatment match for their problems (Depression Guideline Panel, 1993).

If, after the assessment, it is clear that the patient requires a particular kind of treatment in which the provider is not expert, it is the obligation of the clinician to be the patient's advocate and refer her or him to the best skilled provider of those services.

A clinician needs to take the lead in coordinating a patient's medical and behavioral care. As a team member/leader, it is important to clarify which clinician will be the coordinator. In situations involving a psychopharmacologic evaluation, it is important that not only your patient but you, the referring clinician, learn from the consultant the treatment strategy, rationale, side effects, risks, and problematic signs and symptoms of a particular medication regimen. This allows for consistent team work and information sharing with the patient. Also, it is fundamental to consult either directly, with a patient's primary care physician, or to work collaboratively with the psychiatrist liaising with primary care. Information about whether the patient has any medical problems and is on or requires medications is key. These medical diagnoses are listed on Axis III of DSM-IV. It is critical whether your patient's medications may be contributing to his or her depression or irritability.

Medical problems in general—and specifically the very common disorders of hypertension, peptic ulcers, headache, and thyroid disorders—have complicating behavioral expressions. It is important to sort out whether a hypertensive patient with psychological trauma is developing headaches in stressful work with you on trauma and/or has out-of-control hypertension with headaches as the symptom. As well, the related medications in the treatment of medical problems may have problematic side effects which can be expressed as a disturbance in behavior. Steroids, for example, cause a psychotic response in some patients (Gilman et al., 1990). Birth control and hormone replacement medications are used by a very large percentage of women and interact with other medications. For example, oral contraceptives can decrease the metabolism of tricyclic antidepressants, which means that the concentration of the medication is increased; therefore a person who is using such contraceptives can become toxic. In other words, users of birth-control pills should be given about two-thirds the dose that would be recommended for a woman who is not on the pill. The best way to learn about signs and symptoms of medical problems is by asking the primary or specialty care physician directly. This should be part of your normal team-care management. A copy of the patient education materials the physician gives to your patient would be useful for you to include in your records for reference. Your patients should also be excellent teachers about their medical problems if they are treated as partners in their care.

DIFFERENTIAL DIAGNOSIS

Depression is the most common condition treated in the behavioral health community (up to 70% of psychiatric hospitalizations, female:male incidence of 2:1, Weissman, 1987). The etiology, history, and prior treatment interventions—with assessments of their success for a particular individual—assist in developing an appropriate treatment plan. Someone suffering from a chronic pain syndrome, with consequent depression, would have a different treatment plan than someone who has been sexually abused with subsequent depression, versus someone with a bipolar disorder or a chemical dependency problem.

Since the diagnosis and treatment of depression is quite complex due to so many variations and combinations, an algorithm for developing a differential diagnosis and treatment sequence is provided. This is adapted from the Agency for Health Care Policy and Research's depression guideline panel (see Exhibit 4.3).

As you are evaluating your patient and sorting out his or her problems, it is also useful to plan the sequence of treatment interventions that will be most successful.

It is very important to elicit any drug and/or alcohol use, since this is so prevalent, and it is difficult to accomplish other treatment interventions while the patient is still using. The gender differences in choice of drugs, onset of severe complications, comorbidity of other problems such as trauma and abuse, and treatment interventions are profound (Wallen, 1992). Women are more vulnerable to hepatic toxicity, and they suffer more severe complications at an earlier stage in their course of alcohol use.

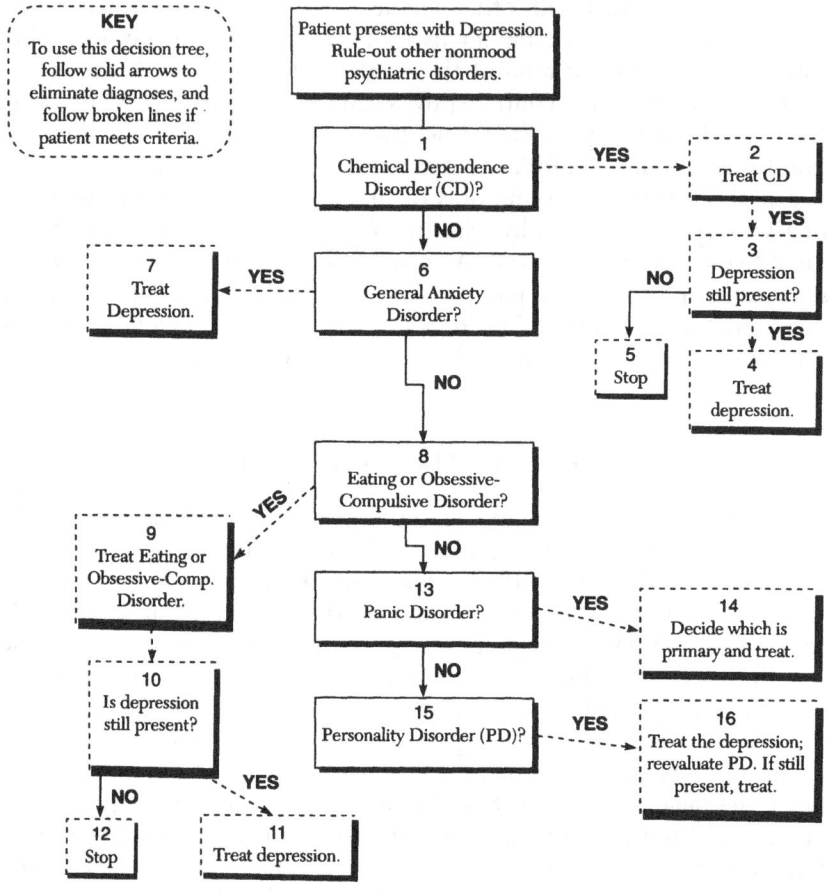

CRITICAL PATHWAY/ALGORITHM
DIFFERENTIAL DIAGNOSIS OF DEPRESSION

NOTES

Box 2:   If depression is severe, both CD and depression may need to be treated simultaneously.

Box 7:   Anxiety usually dissipates once the depression is treated. If anxiety still remains, treat.

Box 14: Primary disorder is described as first occuring, most severity, or family history of illness.

Exhibit 4.3. Adapted from Depression Guideline Panel, 1993.

Anxiety is a more common component of depression in women. Depression may be treated with particular antidepressants that will allay the anxiety as well. Only after this strategy takes effect will one be able to determine if there is a generalized anxiety disorder remaining. Women are more frequently prescribed antianxiety medications than men. Addiction to these medications is still a significant problem. Also, as the patient ages, so does the particular drug used. For example, if a sedative was prescribed in the 1960s, the patient may well be using the same one rather than a safer, newer drug.

Many patients with panic disorder find themselves in an emergency room, since they feel that they are experiencing a life-threatening event, such as a heart attack. Often, part of the treatment approach is a course of a particular antidepressant selected for success in the treatment of panic disorders (Ballenger, 1993).

Eating disorders are common in women, with high prevalence in the college crowd. They are often chronic disorders, so present through the life cycle, particularly if patients are not in remission. There is a high correlation of depression with these disorders. Many women with bulimia hide their disorder. Often their weight is normal. It is difficult to maintain a therapeutic level of medication if your patient is bingeing and purging. Severe anorexia is more difficult to hide. Medication management is difficult in patients with either of these disorders (American Psychiatric Association, 1994).

It has been well demonstrated that certain antidepressants are quite successful in the pharmacologic treatment of patients with compulsive disorders. Severity of illness is an essential component of the evaluation and is very much paired with the patients' limitations of functioning in daily activities. Family members' information on their loved ones' functioning status is crucial. Often the patient's depression dissipates once there is successful treatment of this difficult disorder (Ballenger, 1993).

For many of the DSM-IV Axis II diagnoses, the personality disorders, there are high rates of depression. Depression needs to be treated first and then the person must be reevaluated to determine what functional problems remain. When a person's mood changes, it often allows a new perspective, attitude, and energy to deal with struggles in living her life.

SPECIAL NEEDS FOR WOMEN

Depression occurs about twice as frequently in women as in men due to a greater biological susceptibility as well as social and psychological disparities, including violence. Specific subtypes such as seasonal affective, late-luteal-phase dysphoria, postpartum, menopausal, and oral-contraceptive-induced depression occur in great excess in women.

Until the last decade, a stated rationale for excluding women of childbearing age from drug trials was possible teratogenesis of the fetus if a woman happened to conceive. After three decades of clinical use, it has been demonstrated that this concern for the tricyclic antidepressants is largely unfounded. Since this age group, childbearing age women, has the highest rates of depression and women respond differently to drugs than men, it is incumbent upon researchers and funders to focus on this critical missed population.

Gender differences in drug uptake, metabolism, dose effects, and treatment interventions are immense. Also, the variance of drug effects across the menstrual cycle and life cycle are extreme. For a woman who is very sensitive to a variance in blood levels of medications, it is quite complex for a clinician to provide a *titrated* optimal dose regimen across the menstrual cycle. For example, some women may need an increase in their dosage several days before menstruating so as to maintain their blood level of medication and thus the drug effect. Other women seem to have diminished drug effect at onset or a couple of days after onset of their menses.

The development of different treatment regimens for men and women has been delayed due to the many decades of pharmacologic and other clinical research using men only in clinical trials. It is ironic that women were excluded for so many years because of the variance in response due to their menstrual cycle—the very factor required for consideration in the development of an optimal individualized dosing regimen for women (Hamilton, et al., 1984; Hamilton, 1991; Jensvold, Halbreich, & Hamilton, 1996).

It behooves clinicians to become educated about these issues, since there is a greater percentage of women in behavioral health treatment (Russo, 1990) and a preponderance of women suffering from depression (McGrath et al., 1990).

SHIFTING THE PARADIGM

Clearly, the expectation for providing assessment, treatment, and referral services is precise evaluation and individualized treatment, involving the patient and family in both decision making and the treatment interventions. The goal is to optimize the patient's health status in the most efficient and effective way possible.

Clinicians need to be patient advocates. This includes assisting patients in understanding their health benefits packages and providing service options that best suit their needs. It includes using educational strategies to better inform patients about a wellness model for health. It also includes demonstrating one's own clinical abilities and performance standards by showing how much a patient improves, over what period of time, and at what cost. This is truly a paradigm shift.

The focus on wellness and health, timely intervention, and well-matched services, using algorithms, information systems, and communications, brings in a new dawn for the twenty-first century. It is an era in the health arena of speed, accuracy, and patient advocacy for healthier people. This is an honorable quest. Be part of it.

REFERENCES

American Psychiatric Association (1994). *Diagnostic and statistical manual of mental disorders* (4th ed.). Washington, DC: American Psychiatric Press.

Ballenger, J. C. (1993). Panic disorder: Efficacy of current treatments. In M. V. Rudorfer (Ed.) The value of psychiatric treatment: Its efficacy in severe mental disorders. *Psychopharmacology Bulletin, 29:4*, 487–499.

Beck, A. T., Ward, C. H., & Mendelson, M., et al. (1961). An inventory for measuring depression. *Archives of General Psychiatry, 4*, 561–571.

Brown-Beasley, M. W. (1994). Proposal for a national psychiatric informatics system (N.P.I.S.). *Psychiatric Annals, 24: 7*, 357–361.

Depression Guideline Panel (1993). *Depression in primary care, detection and diagnosis*, volume 1. Rockville, M. D.: Agency for Health Care Policy and Research, #93-0550, U.S. Department of Health and Human Services.

———, (1993). *Depression in primary care, treatment of major depression*, volume 2. Washington: USDHHS, ACHPR #93-0551.

Donabedian, A. (1980). *The definition of quality, and its approach to assessment.* Ann Arbor, MI: Health Administration Press.

Eddy, D. M. (1990). Clinical decision making: From theory to practice. *Journal of the American Medical Association, 263: 2*, 287–290.

Endicott, J., Spitzer, R. L., Fleiss, J. L., et al. (1978). A diagnostic schedule for affective disorders and schizophrenia. *Archives of General Psychiatry, 35*, 837–844.

Fawcett, J. (1994). The treatment algorithms are here, and so is the technology to deliver them. *Psychiatric Annals, 24: 7*, 329–330.

Gilman, A. G., Rall, T. W., Nies, A. S., & Taylor, P. (Eds.) (1990). *Goodman and Gilman's The pharmacologic basis of therapeutics* (8th ed.). New York: McGraw-Hill.

Hamilton, M. (1960). A rating scale for depression. *Journal of Neurology, Neurosurgery and Psychiatry, 23*, 56–62.

Hamilton, J. A. (1991). Clinical pharmacology panel report. In S. J. Blumenthal, P. Barry, J. A. Hamilton, & B. Sherwin (Eds.) *Forging a women's health research agenda, conference proceedings.* Washington, DC: National Women's Health Resource Center, pp. 1–27.

Hamilton, J. A., Lloyd, C., Alagna, S. W., et al. (1984). Gender, depressive subtypes, and gender-age effects on antidepressant response: Hormonal hypotheses. *Psychopharmacology Bulletin, 20: 3*, 475–480.

Jensvold, M. F., Halbreich, U. & Hamilton, J. A. (Eds.) (1996). *Psychopharmacol-*

ogy of women: Sex, gender, and hormonal considerations, Washington, D.C.: American Psychiatric Press.

Karasu, T. B. (Ed.) (1989). *Treatments of psychiatric disorders*. Washington, DC: American Psychiatric Press.

Klein, D. F. (1994). The utility of algorithms and guidelines for practice. *Psychiatric Annals, 24:7*, 362–367.

Lieff, J. D. (1994). Clinical databases. *Psychiatric Annals, 24:1*, 33–36.

McGrath, E., Keita, G. P., Strickland, B. R., & Russo, N. F. (Eds.) (1990). *Women and depression, risk factors and treatment issues*. Washington, DC: American Psychological Association.

Miller, M. J. (1994). A critical review of principles involved in quality mental health software available from computer bulletin board systems (B.B.S.s). *Psychiatric Annals, 24:1*, 9–11.

Radloff, L. S. (1977). The CES-D scale: A self-report depression scale for research in the general population. *Applied Psychological Measurement, 1*, 358–401.

Russo, N. F. (1990). Forging research priorities for women's mental health. *American Psychologist, 45*: 368–373.

Wallen, J. (1992). A comparison of male and female clients in substance abuse treatment. *Journal of Substance Abuse Treatment, 9*, 243–248.

Weissman, M. M. (1987). Advances in psychiatric epidemiology: Rates and risks for major depression. *American Journal of Public Health, 77:4*, 445–451.

Zung, W. W. K. (1965). A self-rating depression scale. *Archives of General Psychiatry, 12*, 63–70.

Appendix

GLOSSARY OF MANAGED CARE TERMS

Algorithm. A clinical problem-solving procedure, using decision tree yes/no analyses, designed by clinical consensus if not based on scientific underpinnings, so that no matter how many times different clinicians apply the same clinical information, there is a consistent, reliable recommendation to apply to the specific situation.

Behavioral health care. This encompasses both mental health care and *chemical dependence* services.

Behavioral health carveout. A type of *fourth party* (see below) arrangement that manages behavioral health using a network of privileged providers without linkage to primary care.

Biopsychosocial. A term used to describe a holistic clinical assessment of a person in which physical health (biology), as well as psychological factors (including mental status, social, environmental, and community context) are given consideration.

Chemical dependence. A term to describe an individual's difficulty with consuming substances such as alcohol, drugs, or other chemicals.

Clinical decision making. The process of analyzing the components of a clinical problem in order to consistently reach the same solution as others and diminish the variance among clinicians.

Clinical protocol. A logically ordered sequence of clinical questions that may be answered in analogue fashion (yes/no) to determine a diagnosis or the most effective, reliable, and valid treatment intervention that will ensure a consistent outcome.

Cost/benefit analysis. As it relates to health care, this is a decision-making process that considers all factors involved in the delivery of services: change in health status, efficiency, effectiveness, cost, time, and risks to patient from a biopsychosocial perspective.

Differential diagnosis. A term used in the formulation of various diagnoses that would explain a patient's presenting signs and symptoms, listing the most probable diagnosis first and ruling out the others, using a logical sequence (decision tree) to confirm or rule out a particular diagnosis.

Effectiveness. In relation to a specific treatment, this is described by the amount of positive change in a patient's health status attributable to that treatment.

Efficiency. The utilization of resources with minimal waste to achieve a given health outcome.

First party. Insurance term used to designate a patient (called a beneficiary of health care services) who is eligible to receive up to the stated health benefits outlined in his or her health insurance contract, based on *medical necessity*. (See also *second party, third party*, and *fourth party*.)

Fourth party. A newer entity than the first three parties, which has evolved over the past 15 years. It refers to the clinical review arm of managed care, distinct from that function which provides services. (See also *first party, second party*, and *third party*).

Managed care. A broad category describing clinical services delivered either directly or indirectly, using principles that consider service quality, effectiveness, efficiencies, and clinical outcomes.

Medical necessity. A poorly understood insurance term defining a beneficiary's (recipient's) eligibility to be covered, up to the maximum of the benefits defined in his or her health insurance contract. If, for example, the beneficiary's policy states that he or she is eligible for payment of up to 20 outpatient behavioral health sessions per year, there must be a clinical reason for those services to be delivered. The amount and type of services are dependent upon the patient's need. The services paid for by the third party are those needed, up to the maximum of the benefit, and not simply the amount stated as the benefit. Therefore, someone who has a diagnosis of an adjustment reaction would utilize only part of his or her benefit, since by definition, this disorder resolves within 6 months.

Mental status. A critical component of a person's biopsychosocial assessment. The key elements to consider in the examination of mental status are appearance and behavior; thought processes (impoverishment, pace, logic, thought disorder, flight of ideas, obsessionality, rigidity, distractibility); thought content (delusions, grandiosity, obsessions, misinterpretations, ideas of reference); perceptual abnormalities (auditory, visual, or tactile hallucinations; depersonalization; derealization); affect (mood, lability, blunting, incongruity, irritability); and cognition (sensorium, memory, orientation, concentration, intellect, insight, judgment).

Network. A group of clinicians who have been *privileged* by a managed care organization to provide services to beneficiaries who have this particular managed care health services contract.

Optimal treatment. The most effective treatment delivered using the most efficient resources.

Outcomes. A broad term that quantifies the change in a person's health status attributable to the health services provided while also considering the resources utilized to achieve that particular outcome.

Privileging. A managed care term referring to a complex process of reviewing the clinician's credentials and clinical performance based on her or his clinical effectiveness and consideration of inviting that clinician to join a network.

Provider group. A managed care term including all types of clinicians who deliver health care services within a *network* or *privileged group*.

Qualitative skills. A methodologic approach to assessment/evaluation in which descriptive statistics are used to quantify variables that are different in kind rather than degree. Examples of these variables include drug use, rater reliability, and occupational status.

Quality management. An organized evaluation system of the quality of care—measuring its efficiency and effectiveness and optimal patient health status—using electronic information systems and the process of continuous quality improvement.

Quantitative skills. The ability to manipulate and interpret the meaning of ordered variables on a continuum where the relationships of equal to, less than, or greater than will hold true.

Reliability. A statistical term used to describe findings that are the same, stable, or consistent when the process is repeated. For example, an intelligence test is described as reliable if a person receives approximately the same scores every time she or he takes the test.

Secondary care. This level of care is more intensive and specialized than care provided at the primary level. It is for those who do not benefit from primary care treatment, which can be delivered by all behavioral health clinicians.

Second party. A term to designate the clinician or provider delivering health care services. (See also *first party*, *third party*, and *fourth party*.)

Tertiary care. Subspecialty care designed to provide the most complex and intensive services available in the field.

Third party. A payor of health care services. The first party's employer group, the federal government (which is the payor of Medicare), or federal/states governments (which pay for Medicaid) are the major third-party payors. Insurance companies are often involved in administering the claims for payment by employer payors. This process is called third-party administration (TPA). (See also *first party*, *second party*, and *third party*.)

Titration. A scientific term used to describe a process in which, for example, the dosage of a particular drug is constantly and carefully measured and evaluated for its effects and adjusted accordingly.

Utilization management. A set of techniques developed on behalf of purchasers of health benefits to manage costs, using a case-by-case method as one approach, to evaluate proposed medical services. See also quality management.

Validity. A statistical term used to describe whether the process being used is actually measuring what one wants to measure. For example, if one is trying to measure a person's level of anxiety, it would be important that the measure assesses anxiety and not depression.

PART II

The Implementation of Managed Care in the Practice of Psychotherapy

The changes brought about by the policies of managed care will ultimately be implemented in the practices of individual psychotherapists, and this is also where the difficulties inherent in those policies will be encountered. In this section, experienced psychotherapists, representing four major approaches to treatment, both express their concerns about managed care and discuss how these treatment approaches fit into managed care systems.

Kenneth Frank is outspoken in his criticism of managed care, but also acknowledges that therapists must respond to the changes that have required a speeding up of psychotherapy. The dynamic and integrative approach to short-term psychotherapy that he outlines is based on psychoanalytic principles, and also incorporates relevant concepts from cognitive therapy. Steven Rosenberg and Phyllis Wright also express concerns about the advent of managed care, but their discussion of group therapy shows how, in many ways, this approach fits in well in a managed care model.

The final chapters, on the systems approach to family treatment by Helen Altman and on clinical hypnosis by William Ballen and Kent Jarrett, share a common theme in regard to managed care. Both of these approaches could fit well into the structures and requirements of managed care organizations, but, as the authors point out, both are little recognized and are currently underutilized by these systems.

R. M. A.
D. G. P.

CHAPTER 5

Focused
Integrative Psychotherapy

Kenneth A. Frank

THE PROBLEM

Writing for *Barron's: The Dow Jones Business and Financial Weekly*, noted financial columnist Alan Abelson sardonically discussed the profit motivation attracting large insurance companies and HMOs to managed care. According to Abelson, "They like it [managed care] because it's so straightforward: Their margin of profit waxes with the population of the plans they manage and wanes with the amount of care they provide." Abelson continued, "The successful HMOs, in other words, are those that have managed to care less" (Abelson, 1994, p. 5).

It is not surprising that a grave skepticism has developed among psychotherapists, many of whom have come to doubt that insurance administrators who are driven to maximize quarterly profitability can also responsively "manage" mental health care. Many providers are understandably disgruntled over substandard fee schedules that neglect practitioners' levels of training, experience, or reputation as gauges of their actual competence. More important, in terms of patient care, practitioners complain of managed care experiences with onerous case reporting that intrudes into confidentiality, threatens the essential continuity of the therapeutic relationship, and involves inadequate and often clinically unsophisticated case review procedures. Significantly, practitioners note that these plans ration services, often promoting extremely short-term interventions that simply are not clinically worthwhile. In the minds of many providers, these objections add up to therapeutically counterproductive ways of managing—that is, *mis*managing—mental health services. From a mental health perspective, the ultimate tragedy of managed care is that it is concerned with procedures and not with relationships, and it is relationships that form the essential foundation of all effective mental health care.

These critical problems notwithstanding, the trend toward shorter treatment, that to some extent antedates managed care and exists independent of it, is inspired by valid concerns over cost-effectiveness. This predictable trend, anticipated even by Freud [1919 (1918)], has been advanced by many psychotherapists who have been interested in modifying the treatment process in order to expand its applicability. Therefore, despite the strong resistance from many therapists, it is likely that this trend will continue, and that it will gain momentum as increasing numbers of patients come under the auspices of managed care programs. In this atmosphere, in which questions about psychotherapy's cost-effectiveness are raised more compellingly than ever before, many practitioners have chosen to oppose all such developments absolutely and uncompromisingly. Others have sought to develop skills that complement their existing ones in ways responsive to the very real and creative challenges framed by the need for effective time-limited applications. The latter strategy, many practitioners believe, will enable them to effectively reach a broader population of patients.

I endorse the position that long-term psychotherapy undoubtedly is the treatment of choice in the majority of cases. However, the current political and economic reality demands that practitioners be able to make the most of short-term treatment opportunities when they are all that are afforded. I avoid further debate of the pros and cons of managed care here; neither do I address specific administrative issues at any length. Rather, my focus is on *technique*. I summarize some of the historical attempts to shorten psychotherapy and briefly characterize the short-term applications of traditional analytic therapy, brief analytic therapy, and cognitive-behavior therapy. Then I describe a shorter-term analytic approach that is synthesized from all three. This approach, which I call *focused integrative psychotherapy*, cannot replace long-term therapy, but can be helpful to a selected subgroup of patients. I have in mind a time frame compatible with that of the more clinically realistic HMOs—approximately thirty sessions.

EARLY ACTIVE APPROACHES

Freud's Observations

There is nothing new about the attempt to shorten psychotherapy.[*] Concerns with the length of treatment developed with Freud, who as early as

---

[*]Most efforts to shorten analytic therapy involve forms of psychotherapy integration. For a historical review, see Goldfried and Newman (1992).

1918, at the end of World War I, astutely anticipated short-term developments when he said:

> It is very probable, too, that the large-scale application of our therapy will compel us to alloy the pure gold of analysis freely with the copper of direct suggestion. . . . But, whatever form this psychotherapy for the people may take, whatever the elements out of which it is compounded, its most effective and most important ingredients will assuredly remain those borrowed from strict and untendentious psycho-analysis (1919 [1918]).

Freud also speculated about shortening treatment by activating the analyst. In this regard, he spoke favorably of Sandor Ferenczi and his experiments with an active form of therapy.

Ferenczi's Active Technique

As early as 1919, Ferenczi took up the challenge of shortening psychoanalysis by (1) prohibiting and/or prescribing certain patient behaviors, (2) setting a time limit for treatment, (3) using "forced" fantasies, and (4) assuming a definite, reparative role with the patient.[*] At pains to emphasize that his thinking was compatible with Freud's, Ferenczi tried to accelerate free association, overcome resistances, and facilitate transference analysis. Ferenczi and Rank observed that strictly cognitive insight achieved through reconstruction of spontaneous childhood memories was overvalued. They stressed that therapy could be facilitated and shortened by experiential aspects of the process—a curative factor that most practitioners acknowledge today. With his work later rejected by Freud and his followers, Ferenczi withdrew his ideas about active therapy in an atmosphere of professional ostracism. Consequently, for many years, further interest in shortening analysis was suppressed.

Alexander and French's "Flexible" Approach

In 1938, working at the Chicago Institute for Psychoanalysis, Alexander and French continued the search for a "shorter and more efficient means of psychotherapy" (Alexander & French, 1946, p. iii). Their timely project, published just after World War II, reasserted that the need for psychotherapy far outstripped its availability. A total of 23 accredited analysts participated in the research, enhancing its legitimacy. The authors' views were

---

[*]See Rickman (1980) for Ferenczi's papers on "active" technique.

similar to those of Ferenczi and Rank in terms of the accent on experiential elements; they also emphasized the need to work through, cognitively, experiential aspects of the treatment process. Stressing flexibility, Alexander and French also placed importance on mastery processes occurring through the patient's deliberate activity between sessions. Most controversially, they introduced the idea of the "corrective emotional experience," which was central to their view. It was based on the difference between the therapist's responses to the patient and the original pathogenic responses of the parents. This approach, fiercely criticized by mainstream analysts (Eissler, 1950), is still regarded as objectionable by many contemporary psychoanalysts from diverse schools (e.g., Segal, 1990; Wolf, 1990).

Alexander and French reported favorable but controversial results. According to Balint (Balint et al., 1972), "had they not claimed that their method 'improved' the standard procedure—which it did not—the heated controversy they aroused might have taken a very different turn" (p. 10). With American analysts so deeply committed to a model stressing the curative aspects of insight, heated debate followed the publication of their project. Unfortunately, the controversy was settled through a further demarcation between psychoanalysis and psychotherapy rather than a reconciliation of differences that could have expanded, informed, and empowered the analytic process.

It must be remembered that psychoanalytic conceptualizations at that time were focused "monadically" on the patient, with the analyst seen as a blank screen. These understandings, emphasizing intrapsychic processes at the cost of the interpersonal, rendered interactive formulations such as those involved in Alexander's therapeutic action unacceptable. Crucially, the prevailing idea was that insight into one's psyche, made possible through a regressive transference neurosis—and not some contemporary interpersonal experience that occurred between analyst and analysand—was therapeutic. Today, in appreciating "two-person" understandings of psychotherapeutic change processes more fully (Rickman, 1957), analytic therapists are in a better position to acknowledge the value of these early contributions. Although Alexander's specific *technique* still remains unacceptable, an overall therapeutic strategy emphasizing the role of the patient's new and positive relational experience with the therapist is thought by many analysts to play an integral role in change processes (Frank, in preparation).

PSYCHOANALYSIS AND SHORTER-TERM TREATMENT

Historically, a segregation has existed among longer-term psychoanalytic approaches derived from the "standard" technique, cognitive-behavior therapy, and brief analytic therapy. It is not only psychoanalysts who have indulged this separation. The bold claims of many brief therapists have done little to promote rapprochement. Davanloo (1979), for example, has caused incredulity among psychoanalysts with the claim that his short-term approach (lasting an average of some twenty sessions) results in *"total resolution of the central neurotic structure of the patient's problems manifested by the total replacement of the maladaptive neurotic pattern with an adaptive pattern associated with cognitive and emotional insight into the dynamic structure of his difficulties"* (p. 21) (emphasis added).

If brief therapy can accomplish so much in so short a time, then why attempt longer-term treatment at all? One answer was provided by Davanloo when he noted that only about one-third of screened patients are appropriate for his modality. Nevertheless, it has been suggested (e.g., Wolberg, 1980) that the majority of patients seeking psychotherapy can achieve satisfactory results short-term and, from a perspective emphasizing cost-effectiveness, that all patients might be viewed as potential candidates for short-term therapy before longer-term methods are undertaken. The time clearly has come for psychotherapists to thoughtfully and seriously explore the ways in which the insights and methods of different therapies can be combined in order to empower their work, especially with shorter-term applications receiving increasing attention.

Even the most liberal among traditional psychoanalysts take a position opposing Davanloo's and assert that brief approaches represent an inherently limited and inevitably superficial way of working. Each of these groups usually makes assumptions that are quite different from the other's. Traditional analysts reject the idea of a circumscribed focus and the high levels of therapist activity that are advanced by brief therapists. There is mounting evidence, however, that analytic therapy, a less intensive and usually shorter-term approach than psychoanalysis, may sometimes produce results that are comparable to analysis in both nature and stability (Rangell, 1981; Wallerstein, 1986).

The views of two preeminent psychoanalysts, Roy Schafer and Merton M. Gill, are reviewed here. Schafer (1973) described a "brief psychoanalytic psychotherapy" lasting no longer than a year.* Rather than deep insight into a narrow focus, which is the usual strategy of brief therapists, Schafer emphasized the benefits of insight into the scope, multiplicity, and complexity of the patient's problems. He described that as the unhurried, nondirective, analytic exploration proceeds, gradually drawing out

---

*Although Schafer originally stated this position in 1973, the recent republication of his work (1992) suggests that it remains his view.

and delineating unarticulated phenomena—including conflict, defense, resistance, and transference—patients ideally develop an awareness of the central role of conflict in their existence and a greater appreciation of their own activity in apparent passivity. Even without elaborate interpretation, Schafer observed, a process of self-discovery occurs with the benign analyst, and a new, organized way of framing one's problems develops that results in relief of the patient's suffering. As there develops a realization that the patient has been active in his or her own suffering, the patient's sense of hopelessness and fragmentation diminishes. A person may reclaim disavowed affects and begin to grasp that he or she may become active in other, more constructive ways that can alter the present, the future, and even the past through active reformulations of experience. Schafer asserted that there can be only a limited attempt in this approach to begin to articulate transference-resistances in relation to difficulties in other relationships. In his view, the termination, though fraught with potential emotional difficulties for both patient and therapist, including their grappling with the disappointment inherent in the limitations of treatment, provides an excellent opportunity to begin to understand the individual's responses to separation in relation to the dynamic conflicts that treatment has addressed. Schafer regarded brief therapy as a preliminary process, asserting that through it many patients may be introduced to a superior, longer-term, and more thoroughgoing analytic experience.

Gill (1984), in a paper significant in that it both revised the author's earlier, influential views of the distinction between psychoanalysis and psychotherapy and also reexamined the psychoanalytic situation in the light of one- and two-person psychological distinctions, took an explicit position with regard to brief analytic therapy. He asserted that what is primary about analytic technique is the analysis of transference (defined as the patient's experience of the relationship), and that this technique should be employed as widely as possible. (He gave the example of a 9-month, once-a-week treatment.) Gill also stressed the value of early interpretations of disguised expressions of the transference in the here and now, as opposed to historical exploration and genetic interpretation. Like many brief therapists, Gill stressed that transference interpretations that apply to relationships outside the analysis have far less mutative value than those directly involving the analyst. Also like brief therapists, he pointed out that this technique avoids an artificial development of a *regressive* transference neurosis. Instead of the confrontational approach of many brief therapists, however, he advanced a procedure attuned to the patient's resistances, proceeding from more superficial to deeper material. Gill's essential approach to a time-limited analysis is the analysis of transference as far as it can be carried.

ELEMENTS OF BRIEF ANALYTIC THERAPY

Approaches to brief analytic therapy constitute a tradition in their own right.° The most prominent contributors to this approach include Balint (1972), Malan (1979), Sifneos (1979), Davanloo (1980), Wolberg (1980), Mann (1982), and Strupp and Binder (1984). Although the duration of such treatments ranges from 5 to 40 sessions, most authors seem to favor 10 to 20. First I will summarize the basic elements of contemporary brief analytic therapy. Then I will discuss how aspects of this specialized approach can inform the efforts of more traditional analytic therapists who are attempting to work shorter-term.†

Patient Selection

While early psychoanalysts who sought to accelerate treatment emphasized the therapist's activity, contemporary brief analytic therapists also stress careful patient selection and the delineation of a therapeutic focus. These authors have specified a range of selection criteria to identify patients who are responsive to their distinct approaches, who are able to engage in treatment rapidly and constructively, and who can then terminate therapy quickly. Some emphasize psychiatric syndromes and psychodynamic diagnosis; others stress personal characteristics, especially motivation. Overall, diagnostic factors appear to matter less than how well an individual takes to a specific approach. Thus a patient's response to a trial run is highly valued by virtually all contemporary practitioners of brief therapy.

Some therapists select only high-functioning individuals. Sifneos, for example, selects patients with notable ego strength and rules out those with severe pathology for his "short-term anxiety-provoking psychotherapy." According to Sifneos, individuals must be strongly and realistically motivated for therapy in order to do well. They must have a good history of object relations, must be intelligent, psychologically minded, insightful, introspective, and curious about themselves. Another favorable prognostic sign is willingness to experiment with adaptive behaviors. In a trial therapy, patients who respond actively, who are able to identify a single focus, who have a constructive response to trial interpretations, and who seem flexible, with a capacity to experience, tolerate, and express feelings, also tend

---

°Under the category of "brief analytic therapy" I include "time-limited" and "short-term dynamic psychotherapy."

† Obviously, I cannot review all of the brief approaches comprehensively here. In addition to primary sources, the interested reader may wish to examine the more extensive reviews of Budman (1981) and Flegenheimer (1982).

to have favorable outcomes. Clearly, these are the same individuals who do well in full-scale psychoanalysis and, possibly, in any form of psychotherapy.

Most other brief therapists are less selective and treat a broader range of patients. Malan, for example, is willing to treat individuals who are not necessarily highly integrated but rules out patients with "complex" or "deep-seated" pathology that may be associated with a potential for psychotic, depressive, or suicidal breakdowns. He also excludes those with gross acting out, substance abuse problems, or unsupportive environments. For Malan, trial therapy must provide the therapist with a clear psychodynamic picture and involve the patient's favorable response to interpretation, especially in the focal area. Wolberg described three distinct "classes" of short-term patients, each with a particular configuration of symptomatic, behavioral, and characterologic features corresponding with different treatment needs. (One such group seems potentially appropriate for focused integrative psychotherapy.) Together with motivation, Strupp and Binder in their "time-limited dynamic therapy" stress the patient's ability to frame the problem in terms of interpersonal relationships and to form a mature, trusting relationship.

The Contract

Early in treatment, most brief therapists establish a "contract" with the patient. Typically, this explicit agreement outlines that treatment will be brief and will be limited to the defined focus. Virtually all brief therapies are implemented once (sometimes twice) a week, with therapist and patient sitting face to face. Otherwise, there are differences in the specific arrangements that particular practitioners establish. Mann, for example, in whose view the termination process always plays a central therapeutic role, specifies the precise number of sessions (12) and the exact date of termination in the initial interview. He initially defines a "central issue" with the understanding that it can be modified as treatment proceeds. Sifneos first states that the treatment will last "several months" (actually, 12 to 20 sessions). Like Davanloo (for whom treatment lasts 5 to 40 sessions), he does not prescribe a precise duration or termination date in advance but clearly establishes the treatment's brevity and focus during the initial evaluation. Wolberg, like many cognitive-behavior therapists, was clear at the outset that therapy requires active effort, including homework, in order to translate insights into action. Wolberg also stressed that the individual must continue with deliberate therapeutic work after treatment formally ends. Some therapists like Mann and Sifneos initially specify that there must be no further contact after the final session. Others, like Malan and Wolberg, permit and even encourage subsequent meetings.

The Dynamic Focus

Following the seminal work of Thomas French (1958, 1970), most brief analytic therapists define and limit therapeutic objectives through the delineation of a dynamic focus. Interpreted in various ways, the concept of a focus remains central in virtually all contemporary systems, since most therapists assume they must narrow the scope of the work in order to assure the most efficient use of time.

The dynamic focus usually involves a formulation about a circumscribed, ongoing adaptive problem, its relation to early experience, and to a historical, underlying conflict. It is responsive to the following question, so important in short-term therapy: "How can one develop a dynamic understanding of the immediate problem that has brought the patient to treatment, that illuminates the most relevant, efficient treatment?" There is virtually no limit to the possible forms that a dynamic focus might take. Based on practitioners' own theoretical orientations and the patients with whom they work, theorists define different problem areas in terms of specific underlying conflicts and therapeutic strategies. The focus may involve any of the following, alone or in combination: a symptom (such as anxiety or depression), a central conflict or developmental arrest, a disturbance of the self-image, a salient interpretive theme, a troubled relationship, or a cyclical psychodynamic pattern (Strupp & Binder, 1984). For Sifneos, the focus must involve a triangular, oedipal conflict. But for Davanloo the focus also can be preoedipal. In fact, Davanloo is willing to address more than one focus in a single treatment. In Balint's "focal psychotherapy" there are "focal *aims*" that are developed from a psychodynamic formulation and serve as a beacon to the therapist in guiding a reparative therapeutic interaction. For Mann, the focus stresses empathy and addresses the patient's "chronic and current pain" related to a negative self-image. For Strupp and Binder, the focus involves a salient cyclical psychodynamic pattern (see Wachtel, 1982). The dynamic focus is framed, according to Strupp and Binder, as a working model or a focal narrative rather than an absolute truth.

Although many brief therapists insist on reaching a clear focus at the time of the initial evaluation, others identify the focus through an interpretive theme that crystallizes gradually over several sessions. Strupp and Binder, like Wolberg, emphasize that refining the focus is the actual work of the therapy. They see the focus as a guiding heuristic that gains meaning and credibility as the work progresses; otherwise, another, more plausible, productive focus may be substituted.

Technique

Although it is possible to improve outcomes by careful patient selection and circumscribed goals, neither strategy is as important as efforts to improve technique. Overall, brief therapy strategies usually include promoting rapid insight into the area of focal distress, helping the patient get in touch with "true" feelings, providing reparative interpersonal experiences, and/or facilitating improved adaptations.

Technique is active. The therapist guides the patient by selectively keeping the work within the focus. In this sense, technique also is directive; giving advice, however, is usually eschewed. Another form of directiveness is a therapist's encouragement of a patient's adaptive behaviors, a technique that traditional analysts tend to avoid. Wolberg, for example, capitalized on cognitive and behavioral elements of the change process by explicitly teaching a "more constructive life philosophy" and encouraging deliberate behavior change. Therapists Mann and Wolberg employ suggestion, too; through a confident demeanor, they promote the patient's hope and encourage expectations that the therapeutic pair can achieve a great deal together in a short time.

As in traditional psychoanalysis, the therapist works with patients' associations, memories, fantasies, dreams, and the like, with the process understood through traditional conceptualizations such as transference, resistance, and interpretation, among others. This material contributes to the therapist's understanding of the patient's psychological functioning, sometimes at profound levels; but interpretively, most brief therapists emphasize the present, pointing their comments toward relatively superficial, derivative levels related to the focus. (In contrast, Malan and Sifneos have pointed out that deep interpretations of forbidden content can sometimes be offered early.)

Transference interpretations, highly valued in most brief analytic therapy systems, are employed both to safeguard the working alliance and to provide insight. Some therapists employ transference interpretations early; others introduce them when transference becomes a resistance. Ideally, these interventions elaborate the connections among the present, the transference, and past experience (Malan's "triangle of person"), relating them to defenses, anxiety, and underlying impulses ("triangle of conflict"). For Sifneos and Davanloo, there is a relentless, confrontive chipping away at the patient's defenses in order to reveal underlying anxiety and conflict. Here the atmosphere is often provocative, tense, and pressured. Practitioners like Balint, Mann, Strupp and Binder, and Wolberg, while also maintaining levels of therapeutic pressure, also tend to emphasize the need for a supportive, warm, and empathic therapeutic atmosphere. Strupp and Binder base their interventions on the "principle of least possible confrontation."

Therapeutic Action

Drawing from the classical model, many brief analytic therapists attribute the therapeutic action and structural change to correct interpretations and patients' resulting insights into their focal conflicts. However, interpersonal mechanisms, especially new relational experience, also play a major if unspecified role in a manner reminiscent of Alexander's "corrective emotional experience." These interpersonal curative factors are conspicuous in the approach of Balint, which promotes new mastery within the safety of the treatment relationship. Davanloo describes how patients often become enraged at the therapist under the pressure of persistent confrontation of their defenses; the therapist, maintaining equanimity in the face of the patient's attack, provides the patient with an opportunity for a new experience of safety and mastery in relation to threatening aggressive impulses. Mann also stresses the curative importance of positive, empathic relational experience rather than interpretation. He believes that patients develop healthy new introjects from the relational processes involved in a successful termination. In the most recently developed of these approaches, Strupp and Binder emphasize the role of both insight *and* new experience as dual mechanisms of therapeutic action. These authors formulate insightful modification of maladaptive interpersonal patterns as a major goal of treatment.

Termination

Many short-term therapists, especially Mann, have concentrated on the topic of termination. Relating this topic to issues of separation-individuation and self-esteem, among others, they have shown how termination itself can become a meaningful focus. In addition to the selection of relatively well-integrated patients who are able to terminate easily, brief therapists also emphasize techniques that inhibit regression and permit the therapy to end fairly abruptly: treatment brevity, high levels of therapist activity, and early transference interpretation. If the patient has loss as a focus, or if there are multiple issues ("foci") or clinical complexities, then several sessions may be devoted to termination. As noted, many psychotherapists insist that there be no further contact following termination. However, others, such as Wolberg, caution that following such rules rigidly can be countertherapeutic; they therefore recommend follow-up sessions. Strupp and Binder recognize that treatment sometimes must be extended in order to work through termination issues.

Post-Therapy Developments

In psychoanalysis, the "working through" process provides an ongoing and intensive opportunity to integrate new understandings with and through a patient's day-to-day activities. Accordingly, working through is usually regarded as a major source of structural change. Since so little working through is possible in brief therapy, how are patients able to change meaningfully? One significant factor involves developments that occur after the therapy formally ends.

In elaborating the dynamic focus, brief analytic therapy enables the individual to begin to observe and understand certain interrelated, maladaptive psychological processes, previously unarticulated, that are both experiential and behavioral in nature. Deleterious influences from the past that shape an individual's maladaptive ways of functioning are convincingly revealed, especially when awareness is achieved directly through the personally significant and emotionally meaningful interchange with the therapist. This relationship also involves an important new relational experience for the patient. Change develops from this awareness, which promotes the individual's recognition of the *active* role he or she has played and plays in cognitive, affective, perceptual, and behavioral aspects of interpersonal difficulties and in the process of change.

From a *cyclical* psychodynamic point of view, conflictual internal patterns, interpersonal interactions, and feedback are all viewed transactionally. With the mind understood as an open system, feedback from new, adaptive actions, sometimes deliberately undertaken, reinforces the development of more flexible and positive attitudes toward the self and others and promotes more adaptive interpersonal expectations. Recognizing this process, Wolberg explicitly encouraged patients to use the tools of self-observation and behavior change learned in therapy in order to continue working actively toward further change after termination. This cyclical psychodynamic view also plays a central role in the action-oriented, integrative approach I describe further on.

THE INSIGHTS FROM BRIEF THERAPY
APPLIED TO ANALYTIC THERAPY

One need not subscribe to any particular school of brief therapy in order to use the insights from time-limited therapies to advantage. Let us consider ways in which analytic therapists accustomed to conducting open-ended treatment might advantageously integrate elements from the foregoing approaches in working shorter-term. For example, because of administrative considerations in a managed care environment, "contracting" receives increased attention. Both patient and therapist must be correctly apprised of the definitions and limits of the patient's coverage. They must understand what disclosures will be made, and to whom. (I have had several patients who have chosen to forgo their benefits rather than authorize the submission of highly personal, detailed information required by an insurer.) There must also be mutual clarity about the goals of treatment, which necessarily become more specific and less ambitious than in longer-term psychotherapy. What will happen if benefits are interrupted prematurely? Will it be possible for treatment to continue beyond the covered number of sessions? Will the patient continue anyway, paying the entire fee out of pocket? Or, if the treatment goals are not realized within a permissible time frame, is it clinically appropriate, and does the patient agree, to have an interval without treatment? Will a referral be made? What will be the subsequent fee? If the specific therapeutic goals are realized, is there an opportunity to continue work on other objectives that may emerge? Under what terms? In a managed care context, it is essential that contractual considerations such as these be appropriately clarified at the beginning of treatment with each patient.

Let us consider some implications of the role of the dynamic focus. Analytic therapists do not always make an active, focused attempt to develop an organized understanding of a patient's psychodynamics. Instead, they may assume an unhurried, reactive role, often even with regard to history-taking, permitting relevant material to unfold gradually over the course of treatment. Refinement of their understanding thus comes about spontaneously and incrementally. If a long-term therapist applies a formulation too stringently, he or she runs the risk of foreclosing potentially productive areas of exploration. But in a time-limited treatment, following themes that do not seem salient runs the opposing risk of diluting therapeutic efficiency.

A reactive, abstinent way of working is often carried over to shorter-term treatments. This approach, derived from standard technique and emphasizing that the therapist reactively follow the patient's associative drift,

is disadvantageous to many patients who are seen relatively short-term.°
The extent to which a therapist follows the patient's lead, permitting the
emerging material to provide refinements of one's psychodynamic understanding, as opposed to the extent to which the therapist draws upon his
or her formulation to actively guide the exploration, is a complex technical
matter. The therapist's organized understanding, providing a tentative con-
ception of the work that needs to be done, forms a dynamic tension with
a more open-ended, explorative approach that is mediated by a respect
for the complexity and ambiguity of personality and of psychotherapeutic
processes. At certain times, especially when longer-term treatment is being conducted, a more open-ended exploration may be desirable; at others,
especially when one is working in a time-limited mode, a more structured
approach often is more effective, in my opinion.

In the light of the findings of time-limited psychotherapy and the growing appreciation of interpersonal mechanisms in the therapeutic action, an
interactive approach and flexible use of a focus appear to be more productive than an abstinent one under the modified conditions of briefer
therapies. Working short-term, the therapist must hierarchize areas of dysfunction and must answer the question "How can I intervene most meaningfully, having the most significant therapeutic impact in the shortest (or
allotted) period of time?" Given short-term capabilities, ambitious goals
give way to more explicit, achievable ones. Short-term approaches require
that therapists participate more actively, including the completion of a thoroughgoing evaluation and history at the beginning of treatment, and regular review of case notes and patient progress in order to more actively guide
the treatment. The validity of noninterpretive, active techniques such as directiveness or suggestion was once disparaged by psychoanalysts (Eissler,
1953), but the role of such "parameters" has become increasingly recognized in both brief and longer-term analytic therapies. Depending on therapeutic considerations, the impact of such techniques on the patient may
or may not be analyzed.

The role of new relational experience has been implicated in the therapeutic action by many contemporary psychoanalytic theorists. It has been
defined in a variety of ways, including empathy, authenticity, and neutrality. New experience has also been stressed by several brief therapists, most
notably by Balint, who understood the treatment in terms of the patient's
attempts at repetition and the therapist's efforts to have certain aspects of
the unresolved past problem "come out right this time, with the therapist
as the replica of important figures in [the patient's] early life" (Balint et al.,

---

°I disagree with the short-term applications of Gill (1984) and Schafer (1973) here.

1972, p. 133). This aspect of new experience is similar to Alexander's corrective emotional experience and also to other, more recent psychoanalytic formulations such as those of Weiss and Sampson (1986). New relational experience with the analyst always plays a tacit role in analytic therapies. Its role in brief analytic therapy has been underestimated.

New relational experience can also be productively related to another important aspect of brief therapy, described by Alexander and French. I refer not to the patient's experience with the analyst that is unlike that with the pathogenic parent but to positive new experiences that occur *outside* the therapeutic relationship and which the therapist's interventions can facilitate. While the direct promotion of behavior change is an objectionable practice in traditional analytic technique, some brief therapists, such as Sifneos and Wolberg, encourage patients to initiate adaptive action. Facilitated behavior change can generate important new material, both interpersonal and intrapsychic, for an in-depth working-through process (see Frank, 1993).

The "foreverness" of open-ended treatment, while promoting an atmosphere in which an individual can feel safe to express and work-through profound issues, can also function in deleterious ways. Long-term therapy can indulge patients' as well as therapists' avoidances related to termination, avoidances that for therapists involve personal as well as financial disincentives to concluding treatment expeditiously. Time-limited therapies, despite other limitations, highlight therapeutic potentials that are associated with the termination process, especially when an absolute termination date is set in advance. Handled with clinical sensitivity, the termination process can consolidate therapy, usefully elaborating the role of issues that have come up along the way. In contracting with patients, a therapist's willingness to remain open to the possibility of extending therapy, rather than limiting treatment to a finite number of sessions, has important clinical implications that must be considered in relation to each individual case. Therapists must be clear about the termination process, how they see its role in short-term therapy, and its potential impact on each patient. It is more important that therapists act responsively in relation to patients' needs than that they rigidly enforce time limits.

The manner in which practitioners integrate the insights of time-limited with more traditional analytic therapies is highly individual. Some may appreciate approaches such as Malan's, with its emphasis on content, accurate interpretation, and insight. Others, especially those who endorse relational points of view (Greenberg & Mitchell, 1983; Mitchell, 1988), may favor the interpersonally oriented insights of Balint, while still others may find Wolberg's approach most congenial. Elaborated in the context of his profound grasp of long-term treatment issues, Wolberg's technique emphasizes cognitive and behavioral change elements in the analytic process. In the following sections of this chapter we will more extensively consider some therapeutic possibilities of that combination.

Before shifting to cognitive-behavioral strategies, however, I would like to note that it is typically quite difficult for therapists accustomed to working in traditional, open-ended forms to switch over to short-term applications. Although one may find that participating actively creates many therapeutic possibilities that a more reactive stance does not, nevertheless it is difficult for analysts accustomed to working long-term to shift to short-term applications. This development is not simply the result of what is asked of therapists in a strictly technical sense. Strongly held convictions and affective factors are also involved. In long-term work, a mutually significant bond of intimacy often develops between patient and therapist. Because short-term work requires the therapist to engage and then to let go very quickly, the therapist often must forego this form of emotional gratification that longer-term treatment involves. Such affective reactions of the therapist, while natural and potentially constructive in conducting long-term work, can create difficulty in the time-pressured, reality-oriented, and pragmatic atmosphere that is characteristic of short-term therapy.

INTEGRATING COGNITIVE-BEHAVIORAL WITH ANALYTIC TECHNIQUES

While many practitioners tend to view analytic and cognitive-behavioral approaches dichotomously, in fact they overlap, and specific insight-oriented and action-oriented techniques can be combined advantageously. In this section, I summarize several specific techniques (cognitive restructuring, self-monitoring, relaxation strategies, exposure therapy, and social skills training) that typically are employed by cognitive-behavior therapists. Emphasizing how these techniques can be employed in analytic therapy, I describe some integrative applications. Then I introduce a focused, integrative approach that is primarily analytic, an approach that has not been widely considered for short-term treatment.

Cognitive Therapy

Because cognitive-behavior therapists are more accustomed to operating with concrete, superficial goals, they typically find short-term work more congenial than do analytic therapists. I concentrate on the cognitive formulations developed by Beck and his associates (Beck et al., 1979) in psychotherapy integration because more than other traditional cognitive approaches (Ellis, 1973, for example), this approach emphasizes an empathic stance that is compatible with that of the analytic therapist. There also exist compatible constructivist approaches to cognitive therapy (e.g., Guidano & Liotti, 1983; Guidano, 1991) that emphasize the individual's self-organizing, meaning-giving orientation, tacit (unconscious) processes, and complex interactional conceptualizations (cognition-feeling-behavior; self-other, for example).

Beck's cognitive therapy is active, directive, time-limited, and structured. The therapeutic model is based upon the assumption that one's feelings and behavior are largely the result of how a person structures his or her world—one's "personal paradigm." This underlying assumption is not foreign to analytic therapists, especially those influenced by Piagetian cognitive psychology (e.g., Stolorow et al., 1987). Yet in many *technical* respects, cognitive therapy can be quite different from the analytic. Therapy isolates and then concentrates directly on modifying "dysfunctional" thoughts, beliefs, attitudes, assumptions, and cognitive processes that lead to distress (such as depression and anxiety) and to maladaptive behavior (such as extreme passivity or phobic avoidance). Like brief therapists, many cognitive therapists focus the work by developing an agenda with the patient at the beginning of each session.

Conscious, unbeckoned "automatic" thoughts comprise the primary data of cognitive therapy. "Dysfunctional" thoughts are understood as negative or maladaptive constructions that individuals make about themselves, their world, and/or their future. These constructions tend to be experienced by the individual as factual representations of reality and are therefore accepted at face value. In addition to their content, an individual's automatic thoughts are understood in terms of habitual "errors" in thought patterns, called "cognitive distortions." Examples of cognitive distortions include overgeneralizations, jumping to conclusions, and dichotomous ("black-and-white") thinking. Dysfunctional cognitions are also seen as signposts that permit the identification, through inference, of underlying, maladaptive cognitive schemas. Cognitive schemas, operating as core beliefs, are regarded as the building blocks of cognitive structure. They are an individual's "rules of life," and dysfunctional automatic thoughts are seen as deriving from them.

One can think of cognitive interventions on two levels: those that seek superficially to modify a person's conscious thought processes and ideation and those that seek to modify underlying cognitive structures. An example of the former is teaching an individual "coping statements" or deliberate "self-talk" for self-calming. The latter approach, "cognitive restructuring," is directed at change at more profound levels and is more like analytic treatment. Let us consider that approach.

Cognitive restructuring is the basic cognitive technique for modifying schemas. The term is derived from the therapies proposed by Beck, Ellis (1973), and Meichenbaum (1977). According to Meichenbaum, it involves

> a variety of therapeutic approaches whose major mode of action is modifying the patient's thinking and the premises, assumptions, and attitudes underlying his cognitions. . . . The cognitive therapist helps the patient to identify specific misconceptions, distortions, and maladaptive attributions and to test their validity and reasonableness (pp. 183–184).

Promoting an "empirical" or "scientific" attitude through a guided examination of the available evidence, therapists help patients test the validity of their automatic thoughts as conclusions. This process of "guided empiricism" or "reality testing," involving "questioning the evidence," is intended to restructure maladaptive schemas. According to Beck and his associates (1979), "The essence of reality testing is to enable the person to correct his distortions. An analysis of meaning and attitudes exposes the unreasonableness and self-defeating nature of the attitudes" (p. 155). A belligerent male, for example, was helped to modify an underlying belief that he must always fight in order to prove his manhood.

Cognitive-Behavior Therapy

Cognitive restructuring can be productively integrated with behavioral techniques. Following the assumption that behavioral modifications can lead to cognitive change and vice versa, this technical integration emphasizes the therapeutically useful interplay between behavior change and insight. For instance, planned "homework" or "experiments" might be collaboratively developed. Consider a patient who holds the maladaptive belief (schema) that she will be rejected if she is assertive. This patient may be helped to attempt to act assertively in a specific situation, and then to carefully monitor the responses to it, possibly in a diary. Such activities help patients to recognize, test, and ultimately revise ("restructure") dysfunctional interpretations or expectations associated with underlying schemas, and to develop new behavior patterns.

Specific Techniques

Let us consider some additional cognitive-behavioral techniques. Although it is not customary for analytic therapists to employ these homework techniques, they can be useful in certain analytic treatment situations, especially shorter-term ones with focused goals, and are capable of potentiating analytic therapies.

Self-monitoring is one such technique. Formal self-monitoring techniques are frequently employed by cognitive-behavior therapists to clarify clinical phenomena and to chart patients' progress. For example, a patient might agree to maintain an ongoing, written record of the occurrence or nonoccurrence of a predefined behavior, when it occurred, where, with whom, and what the patient was thinking and feeling at the time. Diaries also can be used analytically to advance self-awareness and insight. For example, by keeping a diary, one patient was helped to identify the situational sources of his "unreasoning" angry reactions. Another patient was helped to begin to break down ill-defined sources of stress that felt diffuse and overwhelming. Diary keeping can also help patients become more aware of their inner lives and to get in touch with their feelings. By developing a continuity between the work of sessions and the individual's life outside, self-monitoring between sessions can help the individual apply the insights of sessions to "real life" and also provides further material for subsequent therapy sessions.°

Relaxation strategies are used by many cognitive-behavior therapists. These are simple to master; most patients can learn these self-calming techniques in a matter of days or weeks. Although there are a variety of clinical relaxation procedures, in my experience, progressive relaxation training, discovered by Edmund Jacobson (1929), probably has the broadest clinical utility. Jacobson showed that an induced state of relaxation can diminish neuromuscular tension and related reflexive responses, improve mental activities, and reduce emotional reactions. Ever since Wolpe's (1958) development of an abbreviated application of this technique for systematic desensitization, clinical relaxation has had enormous impact on the field of cognitive-behavior therapy. In a comprehensive review of the relaxation training research, Lichstein (1988) observed that the practice of relaxation can be effective in treating a wide range of problems, including sleep disturbances, headache, hypertension, forms of anxiety, and poor anger control. The technique is often integrated with others. Recently, for example, the therapeutic benefits of relaxation therapy have been expanded for the successful treatment of panic disorder through its combination with controlled breathing, exposure therapy, and other techniques (Barlow & Cerny, 1988).† I (Frank, 1990) have provided clinical illustrations of how

---

°The reader interested in learning more about self-monitoring and other techniques reported in this section may wish to refer to Barlow and Cerny (1988).

† The interested reader may wish to review the relaxation procedures described by Bernstein and Borkovec (1973) and by Lichstein (1988), which fairly reflect contemporary practice.

both relaxation training and exposure therapy, described below, can be used effectively in analytic therapy.

Exposure therapy is another widely used behavioral technique. According to Marks (1981), who describes the application of this procedure to phobias, "the phobic is persuaded to enter and stay in his or her phobic situation until he or she feels better, and to do this repeatedly until it becomes so customary that it holds no more terrors" (p. 45). Exposure can be *imaginal* or *actual*. Exposure involving imagery has been called "stress inoculation training" or "cognitive rehearsal"; that involving actual stressors is called exposure *in vivo*. Exposure therapy is often combined with other cognitive and behavioral techniques such as *response prevention* in treating compulsive rituals. Here the assumption, taken from learning theory, is that if a conditioned response to a conditioned stimulus is withheld, its habit strength will diminish. For example, in compulsive handwashing, the compulsive behavior is prevented and the individual is forced to deal with the anxiety that drives it (such as contamination anxiety) in more adaptive ways. *Systematic desensitization* is another combined application of exposure therapy. Here exposure to the problem is gradual, providing an opportunity for the individual to master lower levels of anxiety before taking on higher levels. Other exposure techniques, such as "implosion" and "flooding," are more extreme. Often, as in systematic desensitization, exposure is combined with relaxation training or other methods that are known to diminish anxiety.

Coping and social skills can often be explicitly taught. These include covert skills like relaxation and/or overt skills, either simple ones such as initiating conversations and making requests or more complex ones like negotiating, managing employees, or public speaking. Such interventions have also been used to help individuals manage disruptive feelings, such as anger—associated with a wide variety of situations—more effectively.

FOCUSED INTEGRATIVE PSYCHOTHERAPY

It is widely recognized that insight and adaptive action interact in ways that are essential to the analytic process. It is unconventional, however, for analytic therapists to attempt to directly modify an individual's behavior in promoting personality change. Yet from a cyclical psychodynamic point of view, such an approach is sometimes appropriate, since personality organization, motivation, behavior, the resulting external situations, and feedback all are thought to form integrated elements of self- and field-regulatory mechanisms. In this transactional view, psychodynamic systems can be understood as involving cognitions, affects, *and* behaviors, all complexly interrelated such that a change in any one facilitates changes in other, related personality processes. Especially in short-term applications, analytic therapists might sometimes wish to promote adaptive behaviors in ways that can advance analytic goals.

Through the integrated use of action-oriented techniques, an individual can be helped to examine new behavior patterns and experiences of self; to relate them to the old and explore the origins of both; to compare new and old forms of interpersonal feedback; to examine relationships to transference manifestations; and, importantly, to work through anxieties and resistances, often in the transference associated with the formation of new, more adaptive psychological organizations. In longer-term analytic therapies, analysis of the interaction related to the therapist's introduction of action-oriented techniques plays a major role. But in the shorter-term, integrative method that I am advancing, explicit analysis of the therapeutic interaction may be less important (although the practitioner must always try to remain aware of the transferential implications of the therapeutic interaction). Like methods that seek to modify behavior directly, analysis of the interaction becomes one among a variety of therapeutic tools that may promote progress within the focus.

A *focused* integrative approach can sometimes be highly effective. One useful way of formulating a focus combines interpersonal with object-relations points of view. That is, a working model can be developed that relates problematic interactions and symptoms to rigid, internal symbolizations of the self and of others, including expectations, and their interactions. Such a model relates the individual's counterproductive ways of interacting—to the therapist and to others—to early pathogenic experience and relational conflicts. From such a perspective, understanding, responsibility, and empowerment progress concurrently in therapy.

Focused integrative psychotherapy can have applicability when one is working with relatively well-integrated patients under significant time constraints, especially when circumscribed forms of maladaptive behavior and/or actual symptoms play a prominent role in a patient's characterological difficulties. In the case of one young man, for example, the maintenance of a public speaking phobia was understood in terms of conflicting ties to a sadistic, disparaging father, on the one hand, who undermined his son's confidence and assertive efforts, and to an adoring, worshipful mother who expected too much, on the other. These opposing allegiances, reflected in the patient's conflicted self-concept, were played out in vocational and other patterns as well as the public-speaking phobia and ultimately confirmed his negative expectations. For example, motivated to earn extravagant praise (the tie to mother) and to avoid feared criticism from authority figures (the internalized father), he engaged in inappropriately grandiose but secretive vocational behaviors that finally led to his dismissal from a job. In public speaking as in his vocational efforts, he risked a private, grandiose sense of his capabilities yet felt the conflicting need to conceal himself protectively amid fears of the humiliation of being discovered as a fraud and ne'er-do-well.

It was this overall configuration—the actual phobic symptom, the related maladaptive interpersonal pattern (which became manifested in the transference), and the associated issues of the self-organization—that defined the therapeutic focus. With the therapist willing to form an encouraging but realistic new relationship unlike that with either parent, the treatment progressed on two levels: gradual exposure therapy with relaxation training (stress inoculation) to overcome the circumscribed phobic symptom and analytic work to advance insight into the symptom and the related cyclical psychodynamic pattern. Predictably, the focus came into the relationship with the therapist: the patient related in a glossy manner, avoiding meaningful self-disclosure. When this development was addressed, he was able to reveal his concerns over being discovered by the therapist as an inept patient and thereby humiliated. He spontaneously recalled memories of hiding from his father, who often became unpredictably attacking and punitive, especially when the patient needed his father's approval and support. The patient feared a repeat of his paternal relationship with the therapist; but, ironically, his way of acting to avoid it ran the risk of actualizing the very outcome he feared. In addition to cognitive-behavioral techniques to modify symptoms and behavior, the focused integrative approach facilitated the elucidation of the interaction as it seemed relevant to the dynamic focus.

The authentic new relational experience with the therapist and insight into it are crucially important in this approach. New experience is not viewed narrowly in terms of that with the therapist alone, however. Rather, adaptive new experiences with others, sometimes promoted through the use of action-oriented techniques and integrated through analytic work, are also therapeutically important. In the example, mastery over the public speaking phobia and the related, counterproductive vocational pattern promoted greater confidence and opened up a range of new interpersonal possibilities for the young man. Action-oriented techniques need not be integrated in structured forms; they can also be modified or integrated "seamlessly" to simultaneously explore and promote insight while helping patients behave in ways that serve their needs more constructively.[*]

---

[*]The reader may wish to refer to other publications describing psychoanalytic applications of this approach (Frank, 1990, 1992, 1993).

CONCLUSION

I endorse the position that long-term treatment undoubtedly is the treatment of choice for the great majority of psychotherapy patients. Although concerns about the cost-effectiveness of psychotherapy are valid, most managed approaches to mental health care are inadequate and even can be countertherapeutic. To date, most psychotherapists have found little to encourage a belief that insurance administrators who are guided by an overarching motivation to maximize quarterly profitability can also responsively "manage" the mental health needs of their insureds. Yet practitioners must also be able to help patients in the current political and economic atmosphere, which dictates that they be capable of making the most of those short-term treatment opportunities when they are all that are afforded.

Focused integrative psychotherapy, described here, provides an example of how distinct psychotherapeutic modalities can be effectively combined in a short-term treatment framework that is appropriate for a particular subgroup of patients. Historically, cognitive-behavioral, time-limited, and traditional analytic approaches to psychotherapy have been viewed as distinct from one another. Yet the integration of these modalities can at times potentiate the therapeutic process in ways that are responsive to concerns about treatment efficiency. Although it is not customary for analytic therapists to employ action-oriented techniques, they can be useful in certain analytic treatment situations, especially short-term ones. Focused integrative psychotherapy assimilates action-oriented into analytic techniques to facilitate new adaptations in a way that can extend and deepen the change process within a particular focus. The focus that is defined may include characterological, symptomatic, behavioral, and/or interpersonal (including transferential) treatment goals. Relational formulations elaborate the focus in ways that interrelate historical and contemporaneous relationships, permitting the patient and therapist to understand and reshape the patient's tendency to repeat patterned, maladaptive interactions. The therapeutic action depends on insight, including that into the therapeutic interaction; new relational experience, both with the therapist and with others; the shaping of new, more adaptive behaviors; and thoughtful and sensitive work with the termination process. While not a substitute for long-term care, focused integrative psychotherapy proposes an efficient way of providing treatment to an appropriately *selected subgroup* of patients, and deserves further clinical exploration.

REFERENCES

Abelson, A. (1994, June 20). Up & down Wall Street: Sick cures. *Barron's: The Dow Jones Business and Financial Weekly*, pp. 5–6.

Alexander, F., & French, T. M. (1946). *Psychoanalytic therapy*. New York: Ronald Press.

Balint, M., Ornstein, P. H., & Balint, E. (1972). *Focal psychotherapy: An example of applied psychoanalysis*. London: Tavistock Publications.

Barlow, D. H., & Cerny, J. A. (1988). *Psychological treatment of panic*. New York: Guilford Press.

Beck, A. T., Rush, A. J., Shaw, B. F., & Emery, G. (1979). *Cognitive therapy of depression*. New York: Guilford Press.

Bernstein, D. A. & Borkovec, T. D. (1973). *Progressive relaxation training: A manual for the helping professions*. Champaign, IL: Research Press.

Budman, S. H. (Ed.). (1981). *Forms of brief therapy*. New York: Guilford Press.

Davanloo, H. (1979). Techniques of short-term dynamic psychotherapy. *Psychiatric Clinics of North America, 2,* 11–22.

_____(1980). *Short-term dynamic psychotherapy*. New York: Jason Aronson.

Eissler, K. (1950). The Chicago Institute of Psychoanalysis and the sixth period of the development of psychoanalytic technique. *Journal of General Psychology, 42,* 103–157.

_____(1953). The effect of the structure of the ego on psychoanalytic technique. *Journal of the American Psychoanalytic Association, 20,* 104–143.

Ellis, A. (1973). *Humanistic psychotherapy: The rational-emotive approach*. New York: McGraw-Hill.

Flegenheimer, W. V. (1982). *Techniques of brief psychotherapy*. New York: Jason Aronson.

Frank, K. A. (1990). Action techniques in psychoanalysis. *Contemporary Psychoanalysis, 26,* 732–756.

_____(1992). Combining action techniques with psychoanalytic therapy. *International Review of Psycho-Analysis, 19,* 57–79.

_____(1993). Action, insight, and working through: Outlines of an integrative approach. *Psychoanalytic Dialogues, 3,* 535–577.

_____(in preparation). Psychotherapeutic participation: Interaction, integration, and short-term applications.

French, T. M. (1958). *The integration of behavior*. Chicago: University of Chicago Press.

_____(1970). The cognitive structure of behavior. In *Psychoanalytic interpretations: The collected papers of Thomas M. French*. Chicago: Quadrangle Books, pp. 296–323.

Freud, S. (1919 [1918]). Advances in psycho-analytic therapy. In *The standard edition of the complete psychological works of Sigmund Freud, 17*. London: Hogarth Press, 1953–1974. pp. 159–168

Gill, M. M. (1984). Psychoanalysis and psychotherapy: A revision. *International Review of Psycho-Analysis, 11,* 161–179.

Goldfried, M. R., & Newman, C. F. (1992). A history of psychotherapy integration. In J. C. Norcross & M. R. Goldfried (Eds.), *Handbook of psychotherapy integration*. New York: Basic Books, pp. 46–93.

Greenberg, J. & Mitchell, S. (1983). *Object relations in psychoanalytic theory*. Cambridge, MA: Harvard University Press.

Guidano, V. F. (1991). *The self in process: Toward a post-rational cognitive therapy*. New York: Guilford Press.

_____ & Liotti, G. (1983). *Cognitive processes and emotional disorders*. New York: Guilford Press.

Jacobson, E. (1929). *Progressive relaxation*. Chicago: University of Chicago Press.

Lichstein, K. L. (1988). *Clinical relaxation strategies*. New York: John Wiley & Sons.

Malan, D. (1979). *Individual psychotherapy and the science of psychodynamics*. London: Butterworth.

_____ & Goldman, R. (1982). *A casebook in time-limited psychotherapy*. New York: McGraw-Hill.

Marks, I. M. (1981). *Cure and care of neurosis*. New York: John Wiley & Sons.

Meichenbaum, D. (1977). *Cognitive-behavior modification*. New York: Plenum Press.

Mitchell, S. A. (1988). *Relational concepts in psychoanalysis. An Integration*. Cambridge, MA: Harvard University Press.

Rangell, L. (1981). Psychoanalysis and dynamic psychotherapy: Similarities and differences twenty-five years later. *Psychoanalytic Quarterly, 50*, 665–693.

Rickman, J. (Ed.). (1980). *Further contributions to the theory and technique of psycho-analysis* (trans. J. Suttie). London: Karnac Books.

_____ (1957). Number and the human sciences. In *Selected contributions to psycho-analysis*. New York: Basic Books.

Schafer, R. (1973). The termination of brief psychoanalytic psychotherapy. In *Retelling a life: Narration and dialogue in psychoanalysis*. New York: Basic Books, 1992, pp. 292–304.

Segal, H. (1990). Some comments on the Alexander technique. *Psychoanalytic Inquiry, 10*, 409–419.

Sifneos, P. E. (1979). *Short-term dynamic psychotherapy*. New York: Plenum Press.

Stolorow, R. D., Brandchaft, B., & Atwood, G. E. (1987). *Psychoanalytic treatment: An intersubjective approach*. Hillsdale, NJ: Analytic Press.

Strupp, H. H., & Binder, J. L. (1984). *Psychotherapy in a new key: A guide to time-limited dynamic psychotherapy*. New York: Basic Books.

Wachtel, P. L. (1982). Vicious circles: The self and the rhetoric of emerging and unfolding. *Contemporary Psychoanalysis, 18*, 259–273.

Wallerstein, R. (1986). *Forty-two lives in treatment: A study of psychoanalysis and psychotherapy*. New York: Guilford Press.

Weiss, J., & Sampson, H. (1986) *The psychoanalytic process: Theory, clinical observation*. New York: Guilford Press.

Wolberg, L. R. (1980). *Handbook of short-term psychotherapy*. New York: Theime-Stratton.

Wolf, E. (1990). Clinical responsiveness: Corrective or empathic. *Psychoanalytic Inquiry, 10*, 420–432.

Wolpe, J. (1958). *Psychotherapy by reciprocal inhibition*. Stanford, CA: Stanford University Press.

CHAPTER 6

Brief Group Psychotherapy and Managed Mental Health Care

Steven A. Rosenberg

Phyllis Wright

In increasing numbers, Americans are receiving their mental health benefits through some form of managed mental health care (Cummings, 1991). During the 1980s, participation in managed care programs increased dramatically (Gold, 1991; Hoy, Curtis, & Rice, 1991). By 1990, one-third of all insured employees were enrolled in health maintenance organizations (HMOs) or preferred provider organizations (Gold, 1991). Economic considerations fueled the growth of managed health care as purchasers sought relief from the high costs of traditional indemnity insurance in managed care programs. Zimet (1989) has characterized the changes produced by this shift to managed health care as the industrialization of health care, in which mental health services are managed by third-party payers. The objective of that management process is cost containment—ideally by promoting efficient and effective care. A major consequence of managed mental health care's increasingly large presence has been the expanded use of brief, time-limited interventions in the treatment of mental health problems (Haas & Cummings, 1991; Richardson & Austad, 1991). Interest in brief group treatments has surged in the past several years as a consequence of the development of a variety of approaches to brief group therapy and demonstration that these treatments are both effective and economical. In this chapter we examine brief group interventions and their use within the realm of managed mental health care. This chapter begins with a consideration of the way economic pressures and the need to stretch resources have, historically, shaped the development of group psychotherapy. Next the characteristics of brief, time-limited group interventions are discussed. Examples of the range of group treatments that have demonstrated effectiveness are presented. The chapter concludes with a discussion of the fit between group treatment and managed mental health care.

EFFICIENCY AND EVOLUTION OF GROUP TREATMENT

At the turn of the century, Joseph J. H. Pratt, a Boston physician, designed an outpatient group program for poor patients who were unable to afford inpatient treatment (Goldenson, 1970).

> Beginning in 1905 he [Pratt] brought together groups of tubercular patients and sought to overcome their feelings of discouragement through lectures on sound health practices. He soon discovered that they gained more strength from the knowledge that they were not alone in their suffering than from the technical information he gave them. He also discovered that they gained a spirit of comradeship that transcended differences in religious and ethnic backgrounds (p. 524).

Pratt's assessment of his patients' progress revealed that those who participated in these groups lived longer and healed faster. As time went on, Pratt began to realize the powerful psychological effects of the group's interactions on the individual patients, though that was not his original intent. In short, he had stumbled upon a method that was both effective and, relative to other treatment methods, inexpensive.

The potential of group treatment to alleviate the psychological problems of large numbers of people at relatively low cost is also evident from the early history of the modern mental health era. In the beginning of this century, when Europeans began to explore the various ways "talking cures" could alleviate mental problems, therapy in groups began to be considered. Alfred Adler was probably the most prominent practitioner to use group methods in that time and place (Dreikurs, 1956). As a socialist, he sought to bring psychotherapy to the masses and came to believe that group therapy was the most cost-effective way to do this (Rosenbaum & Berger, 1975).

Other European therapists, also attracted by the potential to treat large numbers at comparatively low cost, experimented with groups in the treatment of sexual disturbances, alcoholism, and other psychological maladies. Thus, from the beginning, therapists realized the value of the group method for treating neurotic and addictive disorders when working with patients with limited resources.

Meanwhile, new group treatment methods were increasing in frequency in the United States. The twenties and thirties saw concerted social and intellectual efforts to develop viable group help models. Intellectual efforts focused on bringing Freudian psychoanalytic concepts—so popular in Europe—to group therapy on an outpatient basis. The evocation of feeling was central to this process. Sam Slavson, a pioneer in group therapy, who worked at the Jewish Board of Guardians during the 1930s, was one of the first to use this approach in group work. The board was a social service agency that ministered to the needs of a poor working class population in New York. Slavson combined psychoanalysis, group work, and principles of the progressive education movement (Klein et al., 1992).

However, it was not until World War II that the use of group therapy as both a supportive and reconstructive technique became widespread in the United States and Europe. The need to treat thousands of soldiers suffering from war-related trauma in a cost-effective manner and the shortage of trained personnel created a crisis of care. Group therapy emerged as a treatment modality that could address these converging needs in the most effective way possible. Thus, group therapy became firmly rooted throughout the mental health world, precisely because of its cost and treatment efficacy (Rosenbaum & Berger, 1975).

During this period, psychoanalytic concepts continued to have a powerful influence in the field. Analysts such as Alexander Wolf and Emmanuel Schwartz were early leaders in this area. They sought to psychoanalyze individuals in groups that met more than once a week. One of the effects of this work was to bring a psychoanalytically oriented treatment, prohibitive to many people because of its cost, into a price range that would make it available to the broader public (Rosenbaum & Berger, 1975).

Economic necessity encouraged the development of group psychotherapy. Group treatment made mental health care available to larger numbers than individual therapy. It is because group therapy is both effective and less costly than individual treatment that its use has been advocated in managed care settings (Rosenberg & Zimet, 1995).

Although encompassing several theories and approaches, to a large extent group treatment has been limited to a single, broadly interpreted theoretical model, namely that of psychoanalytic thought in its various expressions. Consistent with the analytic tradition of depth psychotherapy, most approaches to group psychotherapy have emphasized long-term treatment. Over time, a greater diversity of group treatment approaches have developed (cf. Bion, 1961; Ellis, 1982). However, most of these blended models maintained the long-term nature of group psychotherapy.

Economic pressures are again fostering change in mental health practice, and these pressures are reshaping group psychotherapy (MacKenzie, 1994). The decline in the number of sessions available for outpatient psychotherapy through insurance has directed attention toward briefer forms of mental health treatment. One result has been a remarkable growth in work with brief group treatment and research demonstrating the effectiveness of short-term groups.

Rosenberg and Zimet (1995) reviewed research on brief, time-limited outpatient group psychotherapy for the period 1988 to 1993. The papers addressed in that review were limited to studies of group treatment for adults' nonpsychotic, non-substance-abuse mental health problems. Only studies that utilized random assignment to treatment or control/comparison groups were selected. The studies considered in that review clearly demonstrated the effectiveness of time-limited group treatment. Their review found clear evidence that behavioral and behavioral-cognitive approaches lend themselves particularly well to brief group treatment. In addition, they found that modifications of long-term psychodynamic approaches also provide effective brief group treatment.

Although this chapter focuses on brief, outpatient group treatment it is worth noting that short-term inpatient group interventions have been studied by Klein and colleagues (1994), who report positive results with groups for the treatment of a broad range of disorders.

CHARACTERISTICS OF BRIEF GROUP INTERVENTION

Brief psychotherapy groups share several basic characteristics. These groups focus on problems that are common to all group members; they are time-limited; and therapists are more active in these groups than in long-term groups.

Focus and Membership in Short-Term Treatment Groups

Overall, brief therapy groups are organized around specific treatment goals. These goals determine both the focus and the patients selected for the group. As a consequence, brief treatment groups are constituted with homogeneous memberships. For example, traditional long-term treatment would place a depressed patient who has suffered a recent loss among group members having a mixture of problems and treatment goals. In contrast, a short-term group would place this individual among patients who are similar for having experienced loss. At this point homogeneity is a basic characteristic of successful brief treatment groups (Budman et al., 1994; MacKenzie, 1990; Rosenberg & Zimet, 1995). Heterogeneous memberships are common to long-term groups that are specifically constituted to encompass a wide range of character styles, defensive maneuvers, types of problems, and diagnostic entities. The development of cohesion in such a diverse group requires extensive working through of these differences, which is in itself a length process.

On the other hand, the unitary focus in a homogeneous group provides almost instant cohesion and by its very nature defines the treatment goal (Budman & Gurman, 1988; McCallum & Piper, 1990; Mash & Hunsley, 1993). The focusing on a problem common to all group members allows for an easy sharing of experiences while reducing conflict among participants. Mutual member support is a natural outcome.

Several studies demonstrate the efficacy of brief group interventions for persons having a specific illness, such as genital herpes (Drob et al., 1986), cancer (Fawzy et al., 1990a, 1990b; Forester et al., 1993), and human immunodeficiency virus (HIV) infection (Kelly et al., 1993). Studies documenting the efficacy of short-term group treatment for persons having mental health problems also report homogeneous memberships of individuals experiencing bereavement (Piper et al., 1992), anxiety and depression (Budman et al., 1988), agoraphobia (Evans et al., 1991), obsessive-compulsive disorder (Fals-Stewart et al., 1993), and avoidant personality disorder (Alden, 1989). There were also groups composed of abusive husbands (Palmer et al., 1992) and female incest victims (Alexander et al., 1989). Still other groups were homogeneous with respect to gender (Kelly et al., 1993) and age/developmental stage (Budman et al., 1988).

Length of Treatment

Length of treatment is a defining characteristic of brief therapy (Hoyt, 1990). Length of treatment in short-term groups can vary substantially in duration, from a few weeks to 15 weeks, with the number of sessions commonly around 20 but sometimes ranging much higher. Although the frequency of sessions can vary between once and twice a week, one session per week is typical. Length of group sessions may extend to a full day, but 90-minute meetings are most common.

Duration is an important feature of brief treatment; however, the actual treatment length of any psychotherapy group will be defined by the goals and requirements of treatment (Budman & Gurman, 1988). Budman and Gurman (1988) consider groups running for 60 to 70 sessions as "short-term" (p. 248) when their purpose is to provide effective treatment of persons having severely impaired interpersonal relationships. They define group therapy as short-term if there is a predetermined time limit and the group has a well-defined focus that is treated in the shortest feasible period of time. Although it is difficult to call a group lasting a year or more short-term, it may be considerably shorter than the time traditional treatments require for patients with severely disturbed interpersonal functioning, as is observed in borderline conditions. Perhaps it would be better to speak of these groups as time-limited, not short-term. Ultimately what is most important in time-limited therapy is that treatment is focused and provided in the most efficient manner available.

Budman and Gurman's (1988) arguments for the use of time-limited, longer-term group therapy are consistent with MacKenzie's (1994) recommendation that long-term group treatment be offered to the small portion of patients whose conditions require more extensive treatment. Although the merits of long- and short-term group treatment are hotly debated (Mackenzie, 1994; Mone, 1994) there is little research comparing brief and long-term group treatment. At least some of the research that is available suffers from the fact that the brief group treatment techniques used, at the time the research was done, have been supplanted, in current research, by more effective procedures. For example Piper and his colleagues (Piper et al., 1984) compared short- and long-term group therapy using an approach to brief group treatment that has been greatly modified since that study (McCallum & Piper, 1990). Consequently definitive answers to the short- versus long-term controversy will have to wait until an adequate research base has been developed.

The issue of duration of treatment provided to individuals who require more extensive treatment is far from resolved. Managed mental health care programs generally exclude long-term therapy from the services provided. Often these service limitations are a consequence of a 20-session psychotherapy benefit common to many health insurance packages. For now we can control costs by placing patients who can benefit from brief treatment into appropriate groups while identifying those patients who require extensive services and who will not benefit from brief group treatment. Insurers should be encouraged to see the value of using intermittent and long-term groups as a means of keeping patients with chronic mental health problems stable and thus avoiding costly inpatient treatment (Segal & Weideman, 1995; Stone, 1995).

Although duration is most often characterized as the chief difference between short- and long-term treatment groups, several other essential differences can be cited. A fundamental difference between long- and short-term groups is the nature of their intervention goals. Successful short-term treatment requires goals that can be addressed by a brief intervention. Short-term goals are necessarily clear and limited in scope. Simply reducing the time allocated for traditional, long-term treatment programs is not likely to result in successful interventions. The short-term group's common theme provides a focus for treatment and defines treatment goals—both of which factors have been considered essential to brief treatment (cf. Budman & Gurman, 1988; De Shazer et al., 1986; McCallum & Piper, 1990; Mash & Hunsley, 1993).

Therapeutic Orientation and Effectiveness

The therapeutic orientations of effective group interventions vary considerably. Most of the group interventions reviewed by Rosenberg and Zimet (1995) utilized what Dies (1992) has called action-oriented approaches. These groups make use of behavior therapy (Fals-Stewart et al., 1993) and cognitive behavior therapy (Drop et al., 1986; Evans et al., 1991; Kelly et al., 1993). Other approaches were also represented in the literature. Budman and coworkers (1988) ran short-term groups utilizing an "adult developmental model" (p. 71). This experiential approach focuses on adult developmental and interpersonal issues that arise through group interaction. For this group approach the focus was on problems in intimacy and career, which are common issues for young adults. An approach to group psychotherapy that emphasizes therapeutic group processes and interpersonal learning has been described by MacKenzie (1990). Psychoanalytically oriented group therapy was successfully used by Piper and McCallum (1990) to treat persons experiencing pathological grief after the loss of a loved one. McCallum and Piper (1990) attribute past lack of success with brief psychoanalytically oriented group psychotherapy "to the traditional manner in which the groups were conducted" (p. 433). They find brief analytic group treatment successful when group procedures promote rapid cohesion and have a clear focus, an awareness of time limits, active therapists, and a focus on current relationships and behavior.

Some group interventions used a combination of approaches. For example, Forester and colleagues (1993) made use of support, psychoeducation, interpretive-exploratory therapy, and catharsis in their work with cancer patients. Other group treatments with cancer patients successfully used support, psychoeducation, and cognitive-behavioral therapy (Fawzy et al., 1990a, 1990b).

Certain elements of group therapy are common to all group treatment. In all groups therapists provide support, offer clarification, and focus on core issues or goals, while members share information within the group, and offer support to one another. In many short-term groups but particularly in action-oriented approaches, members set goals, deciding what they will accomplish between sessions. Of course some procedures are characteristic of specific orientations to treatment. Cognitive and behavioral therapies treat patient's problems by changing maladaptive thoughts and behaviors. Techniques identified with those therapies include identifying anxiety-provoking situations, dealing with those problems in hierarchies that progress from easiest to most difficult situations, as well as developing such skills as assertiveness and self-disclosure. Therapists in cognitive and behavioral groups will tend to use modeling and role play to teach skills during group sessions. Members will be encouraged to practice those skills between group meetings.

Treatment provided in psychodynamic groups typically reflects the idea that recurrent, unconscious conflicts perpetuate maladaptive thoughts and actions. Psychodynamic group therapies will seek to help members achieve insight into how their difficulties are related to those conflicts. It is the intent of this therapy to use this insight to achieve a reduction in symptoms and ultimately a more satisfying approach to life.

The Therapist's Role in Short-Term Group Therapy

It is clear that a brief approach cannot be effective if it is nothing more than an abridgment of what is done in long-term therapy. For the therapist trained in open-ended group therapy, the transition to briefer forms of treatment can be difficult, both in terms of technique and philosophy of treatment. The object of long-term therapies is to bring about a major change in character structure—a lasting cure. This is not even conceivable in short-term work, which focuses on using the capacities and healthy aspects of the personality to help the individual advance through life's developmental stages (Zimet, 1979). The role of the therapist doing short-term treatment is quite different than that involved in doing long-term group work. In short-term treatment, the group leader's activity level is significantly higher, cohesiveness is established quickly, and a clear and specific focus on current life situations must be maintained.

Several authors who work within developmental (Budman & Gurman, 1988) and psychodynamic (Piper et al., 1992; MacKenzie, 1990, 1994) approaches have identified a number of important aspects of short-term group psychotherapy:

1. Active therapists
2. Establishing a focus for the group prior to accepting referrals

3. Pregroup screening and preparation of potential members prior to the group
4. Maintaining the group's focus during sessions
5. Group cohesion during sessions
6. Awareness of limits on the group's duration
7. Follow-up after the group ends

Therapists are more active in brief group psychotherapy than in long-term psychotherapy, both in establishing the group and during group sessions, because of the need to attend to the foregoing tasks within a relatively short period of time. Prior to the first group session, the therapist must identify the focus for the group. The selection of patients appropriate to the group is also an important preliminary task for the therapist. Screening of patients is done to ensure a match between potential members' treatment needs and the group's focus and goals. The capacity to relate, psychological-mindedness, motivation, and adaptability are among the personal characteristics that may be assessed in selecting patients for group treatment (MacKenzie, 1990). Activities to prepare patients for participation in a therapy group may also be done to decrease dropouts and to maximize the benefits members derive from group involvement. Once the group begins, therapists are more active because they must work at compressing and intensifying the group processes that, in long-term groups, are allowed to develop spontaneously (MacKenzie, 1994). Of particular importance are therapists' efforts to maintain the group's focus, encourage cohesion, and address issues associated with the group's brief existence. Common to the different brief group therapy approaches is an emphasis upon the therapist's task of maintaining the group's focus on the issues and problems that the members share, particularly the characteristics that guided selection in the creation of the homogeneous group. In the process of focusing on commonalities, group cohesion is also encouraged. Awareness of the time-limited nature of the group is seen as stimulating valuable opportunities for the exploration of members' reactions to change and loss (Piper et al., 1992). Finally, individual follow-up sessions, in which each member can review the group experience and identify what has been learned, can be useful (MacKenzie, 1994).

BRIEF GROUP PSYCHOTHERAPY AND MANAGED CARE

Brief group psychotherapy has an important role to play in a mental health care system that increasingly relies on brief interventions. Short-term group interventions can provide efficient and effective treatment

(Rosenberg & Zimet, 1995). Recently, groups have begun to receive attention as a cost-effective means of providing treatment in managed mental health settings (Budman & Gurman, 1988; Folkers & Steefel, 1991). Indeed, group therapy services are widely used at a number of HMOs. Some have specialized groups for patients with acquired immunodeficiency syndrome (AIDS), incest survivors, patients with chronic health problems, those with chronic pain, or patients with personality disorders (Fitzpatrick, 1992; Folkers & Steefel, 1991).

Short-term groups using behavioral and cognitive-behavioral approaches are heavily represented in the time-limited group literature that demonstrates efficacy (Rosenberg & Zimet, 1995). In part, this may reflect the compatibility of behavioral and cognitive approaches with brief treatment. Behavior therapies have emphasized limited goals and rapid symptom alleviation characteristic of the brief treatment approaches favored by managed care (Mash & Hunsley, 1993). Interpersonal, dynamic, and developmental group approaches have had to undergo greater modification in order to provide successful brief group treatment than have behavioral and cognitive group procedures.

Despite their utility, groups are not as widely used in managed care settings as might be expected. Several barriers to the use of short-term groups can be identified. Among those are therapist practice patterns, whether the patient accepts group treatment, and the logistics of setting up short-term groups.

Certainly part of the problem is managed care itself. Many group psychotherapists, like other mental health practitioners, have found it difficult to make the transition to managed care, with its reviews, limited sessions, and reduced fees. To compound the problem, many managed care firms are unwilling to invest enough effort to help practitioners make this shift.

Dies (1992) surveyed senior clinicians within the American Group Psychotherapy Association (APGA). The majority of the group psychotherapists who responded to his survey identify with traditional group treatment approaches, which are most often characterized by open-ended, long-term groups. Clearly many senior group therapists have little interest in short-term group treatment. It is difficult to know the extent to which senior therapists' preference for long-term groups would impede the use of brief group treatment approaches by others. Since senior therapists provide leadership and administrative support, they could significantly affect the use of short-term approaches by the junior therapists they supervise. Moreover the training that senior therapists provide may not prepare students to use brief group interventions.

Equally important is the marked patient preference for brief individual treatment over brief group therapy (Budman et al., 1988). Potential group members may find the rationale for group therapy less obvious than the logic of individual treatment. Patients may find the idea of group treatment more difficult to accept because it is unclear how they will benefit from group participation. Moreover, patients may prefer individual sessions, where they have their therapist's undivided attention. Groups present members with the problem of forming relationships with others in the group. Embarrassment about their problems produces a reluctance to reveal themselves in a group. The possibility of conflict among group members may be threatening. Potential group members may also reject the value of talking to peers about their problems, perceiving only what comes from the therapist as valuable. Finally, in many mental health settings, clinicians regard group therapy as a less costly but also less desirable treatment procedure. It is very difficult, then, for such practitioners to persuade patients to enter group treatment.

Several steps can be taken to increase the desirability of group treatment. Potential group members can be helped to understand how group participation works and how it can benefit them. This kind of preparation has been done using individual sessions and pregroup workshops (Budman & Gurman, 1988). Folkers and Steefel (1991) suggest a brief course of individual treatment to help patients focus on emotions, self-disclosure, and the introspection that will be needed to benefit from the subsequent group experience. A period of individual treatment can also bring issues to awareness that will be worked through in group therapy. Pregroup sessions with the group leader will prepare the patient for the group by helping the potential group member connect his or her problems with the group's treatment focus. Pregroup sessions can also help patients understand the way in which their concerns are related to the group's focus. Pregroup workshops have also been used to reduce dropouts from group therapy (Piper et al., 1979; Budman et al., 1981). Dropouts decline because pregroup workshops reduce patient apprehension about entering the group. Prospective group members can use the workshop to decide if they can tolerate the group experience. Those who decide to enter the group after a workshop are less likely to drop out than members who enter groups with no preparatory experience. Pregroup workshops can teach potential members skills that will make the group experience more productive. Patients can learn about providing feedback, self-disclosure, and group interaction through a pregroup workshop. Pregroup workshops may also be used to screen out individuals unsuitable for group treatment.

Finally, the mechanics of establishing time-limited groups can present significant challenges. The establishment and maintenance of these groups is more demanding than it is for long-term treatment. At termination, the membership of short-term groups must be entirely replaced with individuals who share problems consistent with the group's treatment focus. To develop such a program, group treatment must be an integral component of the services offered in a given setting. In this manner patients are continuously referred for group treatment as the need is identified, rather than only when a group is forming. Because of these difficulties, only in settings where groups are a clear part of the treatment program are patients likely to be referred in sufficient numbers to make brief treatment groups feasible. Folkers and Steefel (1991) offer administrative and clinical guidelines for the development of short-term therapy groups in managed care settings. They recommend planning a systematic group program that reflects organizational and clinical needs. Administrative support for group work must be provided so that staff are supported in the planning and implementation of the group program. Cross (1995) suggests that groups with as few as four members be constituted in order to shorten patients' wait for groups to start.

SUMMARY

The effectiveness and efficiency of brief group interventions are well suited to the needs of patients and managed care. Brief group interventions have been successfully used to treat a wide range of problems. Their compatibility with managed care is equally clear. Both managed care and brief group treatment require that the therapist keep in mind the importance of setting treatment goals, establishing a clear focus of treatment, maintaining an active therapist role, and working within a defined time span. In an era of increasingly limited resources, brief group treatment remains underutilized despite clear evidence of its efficacy and efficiency. There is little doubt that group psychotherapy can make important contributions to the provision of mental health services within managed care settings. When and if this occurs, however, depends on the ability of practitioners and managed care organizations to make the adaptations that will permit wider availability of time-limited group treatment.

REFERENCES

Alden, L. (1989). Short-term structured treatment for the avoidant personality disorder. *Journal of Consulting and Clinical Psychology, 57,* 756–764.

Alexander, P., Neimeyer, R., Follette, V., et al. (1989). A comparison of group treatments of women sexually abused as children. *Journal of Consulting and Clinical Psychology, 57,* 479–483.

Bion, W. R. *Experiences in groups* (1961). New York: Basic Books.

Budman, S., Clifford, M., Bader, L., & Bader, B. (1981). Experiential pre-group preparation and screening. *Group*, 5, 19–26.

Budman, S., Demby, A., Redondo, J., et al. (1988). Comparative outcome in time-limited individual and group psychotherapy. *International Journal of Group Psychotherapy*, 38, 63–86.

Budman, S. & Gurman, A. (1988). *Theory and practice of brief psychotherapy.* New York: Guilford Press.

Budman, S., Simone, P., Reilly, R., & Demby, A. (1994). Progress in short-term and time-limited group psychotherapy: Evidence and implications. In A. Fuhriman & G. Burlingame (Eds.), *Handbook of group psychotherapy: An empirical and clinical synthesis.* New York: Wiley.

Cross, C. D. (1995). Organizing group psychotherapy programming in managed care settings. In K. R. MacKenzie (Ed.) *Effective use of group therapy in managed care.* Washington, DC: American Psychiatric Press.

Cummings, N. (1991). Arguments for the financial efficacy of psychological services in health care settings. In J. Sweet, R. Rozensky, & S. Tovian (Eds.), *Handbook of clinical psychology in medical settings* (pp. 113–126). New York: Plenum Press.

Dreikurs, R. (1956). The contribution of group psychotherapy to psychiatry. *Group Psychotherapy*, 9, 115–125.

De Shazer, S., Berg, I., Lipchik, E., et al. (1986). Brief therapy: Focused solution development. *Family Process*, 25, 207–222.

Dies, R. (1992). Models of group psychotherapy: Sifting through confusion. *International Journal of Group Psychotherapy*, 42, 1–17.

Drob, S., Bernard, H., Lifshutz, H., & Nierenberg, A. (1986). Brief group psychotherapy for Herpes patients: A preliminary study. *Behavior Therapy*, 17, 229–238.

Ellis, A. (1982). Rational-emotive group therapy. In G. M. Gazda (Ed.). *Basic approaches to group psychotherapy and group counseling*, 3rd ed. (pp. 381–412). Springfield, IL: Charles C. Thomas.

Evans, L., Holt, C., & Oei, T. (1991). Long-term follow-up of agoraphobics treated by brief intensive group cognitive behavioural therapy. *Australian and New Zealand Journal of Psychiatry*, 25, 343–349.

Fals-Stewart, W., Marks, A., & Schafer, J. (1993). A comparison of behavioral group therapy and individual behavior therapy in treating obsessive-compulsive disorder. *Journal of Nervous and Mental Disease*, 181, 189–193.

Fawzy, F., Counsins, N., Fawzy, N., et al. (1990a). A structured psychiatric intervention for cancer patients: I. Changes over time in methods of coping and affective disturbance. *Archives of General Psychiatry*, 47, 720–725.

Fawzy, F., Kemeny, M., Fawzy, N., et al. (1990b). A structured psychiatric intervention for cancer patients: II. Changes over time in immunological measures. *Archives of General Psychiatry*, 47, 729–735.

Fitzpatrick, R. (1992). The Harvard Community Health Plan: An evolving model of managed mental health care. In J. Feldman & R. Fitzpatrick (Eds.), *Managed mental health care: Administrative and clinical issues* (pp. 385–399). Washington, DC: American Psychiatric Press.

Folkers, C., & Steefel (1991). Group psychotherapy. In C. Austad & W. Berman (Eds.), *Psychotherapy in managed care: The optimal use of time and resources* (pp. 46–64). Washington, DC: American Psychological Association.

Forester, B., Kornfeld, D., Fleiss, J., & Thompson, S. (1993). Group psychotherapy during radiotherapy: Effects on emotional and physical distress. *American Journal of Psychiatry, 150,* 1700–1706.

Gold, M. (1991). HMOs and managed care. *Health Affairs, 10,* 189–206.

Goldenson, R. (1970). *The encyclopedia of human behavior,* vol. 1. Garden City, NY: Doubleday.

Haas, L., & Cummings, N. (1991). Managed outpatient mental health plans: Clinical, ethical, and practical guidelines for participation. *Professional Psychology: Research and Practice, 22,* 45–51.

Hoy, E., Curtis, R., & Rice, T. (1991). Change and growth in managed care. *Health Affairs, 10,* 18–36.

Hoyt, M. (1991). On time in brief therapy. In R. Wells & V. Giannetti (Eds.) *Handbook of the Brief Psychotherapies.* New York: Plenum Press.

Kelly, J., Murphy, D., Bahr, R., et al. (1993). Outcome of cognitive-behavioral and support group brief therapies for depressed, HIV infected persons. *American Journal of Psychiatry, 150,* 1679–1686.

Klein, R., Bernard, H., Singer, D. (Eds.) (1992). *Handbook of contemporary group psychotherapy* (pp. 1–27). Madison, CT: International Universities Press.

Klein, R., Brabender, V., & Fallon, A. (1994). Inpatient group therapy. In A. Fuhriman & G. Burlingame (Eds.), *Handbook of group psychotherapy: An empirical and clinical synthesis.* New York: Wiley.

MacKenzie, K. R. (1990). *Introduction to time-limited group psychotherapy.* Washington, DC: American Psychiatric Association Press.

MacKenzie, K. R. (1994). Where is here and when is now? The adaptational challenge of mental health reform for group psychotherapy. *International Journal of Group Psychotherapy, 44,* 407–428.

Mash, E., & Hunsley, J. (1993). Behavior therapy and managed mental health care: Integrating effectiveness and economics in mental health practice. *Behavior Therapy, 24,* 67–90.

McCallum, M., & Piper, W. (1990). A controlled study of effectiveness and patient suitability for short-term group psychotherapy. *International Journal of Group Psychotherapy, 40,* 431–452.

Mone, L. (1994). Managed care cost effectiveness: Fantasy or reality. *International Journal of Group Psychotherapy, 44,* 437–448.

Palmer, S., Brown, R., & Barrera, M. (1992). Group treatment for abusive husbands: Long-term evaluation. *American Journal of Orthopsychiatry, 62,* 276–283.

Piper, W., Debbane, E., Garant, J., & Bienvenu, J. (1979). Pretraining for psychotherapy: A cognitive-experiential approach. *Archives of General Psychiatry, 36,* 1250–1256.

Piper, W., Debbane, E., Bienvenu, J., & Garant, J. (1984). A comparative study of four forms of psychotherapy. *Journal of Consulting and Clinical Psychology, 52,* 268–279.

Piper, W., McCallum, M., & Azim, H. (1992). *Adaptation to loss through short-term group therapy*. New York: Guilford Press.

Richardson, L., & Austad, C. (1991). Realities of mental health practice in managed-care settings. *Professional Psychology: Research and Practice, 22*, 52–59.

Rosenbaum, M., & Berger, M. (1975). Introduction. In Rosenbaum, M. & Berger, M. (Eds.) *Group psychotherapy and group functions—Revised*. New York: Basic Books.

Rosenberg, S., & Zimet, C. (1995). Brief group treatment and managed mental health care. *International Journal of Group Psychotherapy, 45*, 367–379.

Segal, B., & Weideman, R. (1995). Outpatient groups for patients with personality disorders. In K. R. MacKenzie (Ed.). *Effective use of group therapy in managed care*. Washington, DC: American Psychiatric Press.

Stone, W. (1995). Group therapy for seriously mentally ill patients in a managed care system. In K. R. MacKenzie (Ed.). *Effective use of group therapy in managed care*. Washington, DC: American Psychiatric Press.

Zimet, C. (1979). Developmental task and crises groups: An application of group psychotherapy to maturational processes. *Psychotherapy: Theory, Research and Practice, 16*, 2–8.

Zimet, C. (1989). The mental health care revolution: Will psychology survive? *American Psychologist, 44*, 704–708.

CHAPTER 7

Family Systems Therapy: Meeting the Challenge of Managed Care

Helen Altman

As the challenges of managed care's restrictiveness become more pervasive, this therapist believes that using a family systems model of therapy* can prove beneficial for patient care and at the same time be compatible with many of the goals of health care management.

A brief overview of the literature is intended to help the reader make the transition to the beginnings of the family therapy movement, even as the halcyon days of Freudian theory were also adding new disciples. Some of the basic tenets of systems thinking are illustrated with case vignettes from the author's practice, which should be helpful to the reader who may be less familiar with this approach.

At the same time, the context in which managed care has evolved is examined. Although there are many compatibilities with family systems therapy, the newer, more stringent approaches taken by many of these companies are, to this therapist's thinking, erroneous, given what we know today about diagnostic predictability and relational diagnoses and may be detrimental to good patient care. These issues are also discussed in the second section.

---

*We include all those trained in marriage and family therapy who, regardless of differences in approach, acknowledge the "common thread" of "the influence of general systems theory" (Kaslow, 1996, p. 7).

BACKGROUND LITERATURE

"The family is basic to human experience. It is the primary social context that shelters the infant, nourishes the child, guides the youth, cradles the love of man and woman, and protects the old. The family eases us into life, and, finally, eases our departure from it. The central importance of family is part of our shared wisdom" (Ackerman Institute for Family Therapy, current brochure). As early as 1937, Nathan Ackerman, trained in psychoanalysis, yet a pioneer in family therapy wrote, "None of us live our lives entirely alone. . . . we live our lives with others; our adjustments to life are in the greatest measure determined by the contingencies of our interpersonal relationships" (Ackerman, 1982, p. 153).

Ackerman's understanding of family relationships developed from the child guidance movement. However, following World War II, a major impetus toward a family perspective came from "failures" within the mainstream of psychiatric understanding with two distinct populations, namely, schizophrenics and their families and delinquent and poor children.

During the 1950s, efforts increased to involve the family in the therapy of the patient, because many psychiatrists whose patients had been "cured" in the hospital and then discharged home to their families had seen these patients relapse or develop exacerbated symptoms. As clinicians and researchers began to accept the importance of the family to the clinical situation, the "shifting focus from individual to family confronted these investigators with the dilemma of describing and conceptualizing a family relationship system" (Kerr, 1981, p. 228).

Murray Bowen's pursuit of the etiology of schizophrenia expanded the development of a family systems theory. He first hospitalized mothers with their schizophrenic children and later shifted his research by hospitalizing the entire family unit. The emergence of family therapy, and the formulation of a theory evolved from this early research. Bowen's emphasis was on the family of origin, the impact of "triangulation" within the family system, and of a multigenerational transmission of beliefs and myths, spoken or not, that permeate several generations of the family.

As these ideas began to circulate, smaller studies focused on family interactional patterns when hospitalized patients went home. One such study (Altman-Jacobs, 1958) examined the impact on family relationships of hospitalized children, who by research design returned home on the weekends to be with their parents. The contrast between the childrens' behavior in the hospital compared to home was impressive.

In contrast to Bowen, "the southern gentleman," Salvador Minuchin, born to Russian-Jewish emigrants in Argentina, "has been guided by a sense of social purpose in a way that has set him apart from the other figures who have shaped family therapy" (Simon, 1984, p. 22). In his dramatic work at the Wiltwick School (Minuchin et al., 1967), a therapeutic approach developed that was founded on the immediacy of the present reality, was oriented to solving problems, and was above all contextual (Aponte & Van Deusen, 1981, p. 310) meaning that the social environment which was impoverished was uniquely part of the problems these families faced. In the development of his work, structural family therapy, it should not be too surprising that the notions about hierarchy, boundaries, and subsystems sprang from these beginnings.

Although ethnicity, culture, and poverty are not a focus of this chapter, it would be well for the reader to reflect upon the significance of the manner in which these attributes affect our own personal sense of therapy and reaffirm the context within which the patient lives and functions.

By the late 1970s, the deinstitutionalization movement, on behalf of the chronically mentally ill became a reality. Many of these patients were being discharged back to their families who had little experience in coping with such severe illness. Additionally, blame by the mental health establishment for causing the illness, or those who believed that the illness "served a function" in the family system (Terkelsen, 1983) created an intense backlash which led to the proliferation of psychoeducational programs for the family. (Anderson, Hogarty, & Reiss, 1980; Falloon & Liberman, 1983; Frances, Clarkin, & Perry, 1984; Hogarty et al., 1986; McFarlane et al., 1995).

At this point, some of the significant differences between traditional individual psychotherapy and family systems therapy should be addressed. The former views mental problems as located within an individual, that is, symptomatology is assumed to be due to a dysfunction within the individual. By contrast, family therapists are not interested in whether the family produced pathology in an individual, but rather focus on how family members *respond* to the so-called "pathological" behavior and what seems to perpetuate the individual's symptomatic functioning within the family system.

In her seminal work, Peggy Papp offers her approach to this work. "The key concepts of systems thinking have to do with wholeness, organization, and patterning. . . . This concept of patterning and circular organization, as opposed to individual description and linear explanation, has become the foundation upon which family therapy rests" (Papp, 1983, p. 7).

Some of the latest research to emerge is "a convincing body of scientific evidence supporting the efficacy of marriage and family therapy." (*Journal of Marital and Family Therapy*, 1995, p. 610). This special issue, titled "The Effectiveness of Marital and Family Therapy" describes research and outcome studies for such diverse diagnostic categories as affective disorders, disorders of childhood and adolescents, alcohol and drug addictions, and the treatment of physical and mental illness. Much of the research supports earlier findings by Simmons and Doherty (1995), which demonstrate "that marriage and family therapy deals with a broad range of mental health problems similar to the practice of other mental health professionals, is relatively brief compared to the other forms of intervention, and is also more cost effective" (Sprenkle & Bailey, 1995, p. 339).

What a wonderful affirmation for the benefit of our patients facing the challenges of managed care!

WORKING WITHIN A SYSTEMS PERSPECTIVE

"The assumptions of family systems therapy are based on the idea that the family is the primary and, except in rare circumstances, the most powerful emotional system we ever belong to, which shapes and continues to determine the course and outcome of our lives" (Silverstein, 1984, p. 3). Most likely, all clinicians would agree that we are in large part dealing with the impact of the original family and how it has shaped our relationships in present situations. Milton Erickson puts it succinctly: "Psychotherapy is sought not primarily for enlightenment about the unchangeable past but because of dissatisfaction with the present and a desire to better the future" (Erickson, 1974, Foreword). The difference is how we as therapists choose to handle the patient's request for help with the information that is initially presented to us. As an illustration, the reader is encouraged to review a psychoanalytic approach (Alperin, 1994) and a systems approach to the same case (Altman, 1995), which under managed care, treatment was limited to 20 sessions.

Family systems therapy has to do with how one *thinks*. It is a profoundly different way of conceptualizing a presenting problem, knowing what questions to ask that will elicit the information needed for sound clinical judgment without the need to pathologize the patient, family, or situation. Systems theory does not have to abbreviate its rationale just to "fit in" with managed care criteria. Just as brief, focused therapy is not merely an abbreviated form of long-term therapy, so too systems therapy is more than how many family members, single or multiple, may be sitting in the therapist's office at the same time. As the technology in our field continues to develop in working effectively within a relatively short time, an easier relationship (not alliance) can be forged with managed care.

With a family systems approach, the therapy is informed by the context in which a patient has lived and is functioning. This perspective is based on a model of change in behavior and functioning (which *then* brings forth the feelings connected to these events), not insight or intrapsychic phenomena.

As one observes the circular nature of interactions and reciprocity of responses within a family ("*He* always says that," "*She's* the shy one," etc.), the usefulness of a cause-and-effect explanation seem to vanish. Rather, the therapy is an active participatory process between therapist and client, couple, or family that focuses on the who, what, where, when, and how, in order to elicit the reciprocal and repetitive patterns and interaction between family members. Tasks are given as thinking and planning exercises: how they are carried out or not gives information regarding functioning rather than "motivational" or "resistance" judgments about the patient or family. The dilemma of the need to change and at the same time, the wish to remain the same is the precarious position in which patients find themselves when they seek help. Regardless of the number of people involved in the session, the emotional issues and expressions of feeling that emerge are directed back to the natural relationships rather than brought into the therapy sessions as transference. Because of this, termination has more to do with what has or has not been accomplished, with less emphasis on the disengagement process between patient and therapist.

One of the hardest tasks initially is to develop with a patient a problem definition that is goal-oriented and "possible." By "possible," we mean arriving at a mutual understanding of where the patient seems stuck, or is most unhappy in life at this particular time, so that a shared perception can develop in order to define the problem in such a way that will open up the opportunity for change. "Possible" also means, in the world of managed care, "do-able"—that is, what can be accomplished within a certain number of sessions that is compatible with the *mutual understanding* upon which the patient and the therapist have agreed. For example:

> The White family was referred by the father's psychiatrist because of frequent arguments and occasional violence between the parents with consequent disruptions in their three adolescents' lives in school and on vacation. Although the father had been in private therapy for many years, family acceptance of this referral was that it would stop the fights, control the father's drinking, and make them a "loving, happy family" again.
>
> However, at the initial session, the therapist observed that patterns of communication which emerged between family members represented long-standing and complicated relationships in which blame was widespread and no consensus could be reached as to who or what the problem was. The therapist wondered if the daughter's forthcoming Confirmation, which had a specific date within the managed care limit, could become the focal point for therapy. However, this clinical decision could be made regard-

less of the method of reimbursement, private pay or managed care. This move allowed family members to take responsibility for his/her individual behavior as it related to the anticipated family celebration, and also set a time frame which for them seemed possible and which could be tolerated without the risk of dropping out of treatment.

At the same time, an intervention frequently used by strategic therapists, predicting regression as the therapy is ending, was given to underscore the dilemma of stability and change. This therapist reminded the family that having experienced some calm in their lives instead of chaos, they could now make an "informed" choice as to what their behavior could be in the future. A follow-up letter from the father stated "no fights amongst our family . . . peace and tranquility reigned supreme." Course of treatment: 11 sessions over 5 months.

One of the techniques frequently used in systems work is that of reframing. "Reframing or providing an alternative explanation about behavior" (Riché-Ault, 1983, p. 68) can allow a shift in the patient's perspective of what went "wrong," thus creating a new construct that offers the opportunity for new behavior to emerge. It is not so much the patient's "reality" as it is the *perception* the patient holds about family, social, or work life and the stories that flow from these experiences which are useful for therapeutic intervention. As a different, more positive "sense of self" is experienced, the patient becomes less interested in retelling the old, time-consuming stories, thus shortening the course of treatment.

Hedda, a successful business woman of Hispanic background, sought treatment when her married daughter Nellie divorced her husband during pregnancy. Because Hedda had divorced Nellie's father when the daughter was two, living away from family and on welfare, she saw Nellie's current behavior as following in her footsteps, indicating her failure as a mother. When it was suggested that perhaps Nellie's view of that time was different, that she saw her mother as courageous and with an ability to function independently, Hedda began to accept that what she had recalled as utter misery, her daughter saw as qualities of strength. This shift in perception diminished her anxiety about the forthcoming birth and allowed a reconciliation between the two women. Course of treatment: 12 sessions over 8 months.

Another technique used in therapy is the way in which family history, often elicited by the use of a genogram, can be useful. The importance of a three-generational history is to help illuminate the family's own belief system about events, relationships, and behavior which have passed down from generation to generation. Information is sought as it is relevant to the presenting problem, thus eliminating what might take several sessions for nonessential history gathering. What Bowen (1976) called the "multigenerational transmission" process is illustrated by the following.

> John and his wife, both middle-aged and recently married, were referred by their employee assistance program (EAP) for counseling following the birth of their daughter because of severe disagreements over his and her financial responsibilities; John's continuing physical complaints, which his wife viewed as hypochondriacal; and their polarized views about child care. For example, his wife's laid back attitude toward the baby's colds, coughs, and crying in the night were countered by John's almost hysterical level of concern about the baby and the need to call the pediatrician immediately. John himself was terrified that should he be left alone with the baby, he might die of a heart attack. What seemed to be his reluctance to baby-sit and do other chores around the house had its own unique connections in the past.
> A three-generational genogram revealed that John's father and mother each had suffered an early parental death, and that these early losses seemed to be transmitted through family members by extreme closeness, both emotionally and financially. John was encouraged to set a personal goal of what *he* would be doing when his daughter was beyond the critical age. Subsequently, his chest pains subsided.

Such an example illustrates the effects of past trauma, and, although known as historical fact, how it is transmitted multigenerationally with profound emotional impact on the current situation. Additionally, what an interesting dilemma to highlight gender attitudes and their effect on therapy. As a woman, this author was initially more empathic with the wife's complaints about undone household chores. Yet a male therapist might have aligned himself with John's reluctance for "domestic" chores, (perhaps even wondering if John's anxiety about physical ailments might be a part of it). Acceptance of either position would have been an error, because they stem from the still prevailing patriarchal model of the family in which roles are supposed to be complementary, that is, the male as wage earner and the woman in charge of the emotional tone of the home. Within a feminist model of therapy, each partner would be responsible for both financial stability and emotional expressiveness, a more symmetrical position. (Walters et al., 1988).

Regardless of the number of the people in the session or therapy, the therapist continues to actively engage the patient's thinking and reaction to the other person(s). "What did you *do* when he canceled plans because of a business trip" instead of "how did that make you feel" offers the idea that a patient can respond differently, which, in turn, may alter the prior feelings (possibly of rejection). "From doing something different comes different thinking and feeling" (Weakland, in Wylie, 1990, p. 33), thus moving the therapy along at a faster pace. If the reader thinks we are being disrespectful regarding a patient's feelings by inquiring about behavior, ask a friend or neighbor "What did you *do* when you went to the PTA meeting which was canceled without warning?" Any one of us will hear the story out and know exactly how our friend *felt* about the situation.

> Penny, age 34, entered treatment because the relationship with her current boyfriend had the uncomfortable characteristics of previous involvements, including a failed marriage. She described an on-again/off-again style which we agreed had the qualities of a pursuer/distancer romance. As she described the sequence, I asked if she thought her boyfriend would see it the same way. Once she became aware of her behavior within the cycle, I then asked if she was aware of what triggered her boyfriend's vacillating behavior. "If he were sitting here with us, how do you think he would answer?" The speculative questions about the "other person" helped her understand the reciprocal patterns within the relationship so that she could begin to diminish her cue-inducing behavior, thereby becoming more in charge of herself and less a victim of circumstance.

For the trained systems therapist, the work offers an opportunity for elegance and efficiency in helping people with problems. For this therapist, like many who have been trained in psychoanalytical or psychodynamic psychotherapy, the shift in thinking and focus was initially difficult, yet it was also exhilarating and fresh.

THE DEVELOPMENT OF A TENTATIVE HYPOTHESIS WITHIN A FAMILY SYSTEMS THERAPY FRAMEWORK

The following material is from the first interview with a depressed patient whose course of treatment was 9 sessions over 5 months.

Carol, a 22-year-old black, obese woman, was referred by the EAP from a local business where she held an internship for 6 months from college, located in another state. Her supervisor became concerned with Carol's apparent sadness, particularly as she knew that Carol was living alone at the YWCA and seemed unable to form any social connections. Her insurance, under managed care, authorized 10 sessions.

At our first session, Carol, whose parents are middle-class college graduates, said she has always felt like "the black sheep" of the family. Her older brother had graduated from college, was engaged to be married 7 months hence, and lived away from home. The family had moved several times cross country for the father's jobs and she acknowledged her difficulties over the years in making new friends in a variety of different school settings.

Her father frequently had job crises and bouts of unemployment as an executive. Nevertheless, at the time Carol was about to depart for college, he assured his daughter, as he had done previously with his son, that even if he had to "sell the family home," he would put them through school. Carol described her mother as rather snobbish, someone whose social friends were more often white, paying great attention to what she herself later described as the "social niceties." Carol had known for many years about her mother's unhappiness in the marriage. Her mother frequently told her that she planned to divorce as soon as Carol graduated from college.

Carol had selected a college with a work/study program away from home, but after several months found herself becoming quite unhappy, often calling her mother. Determined not to quit, she had 2 years of counseling at college, during which time her mother called the counselor frequently, wanting to know what was happening in therapy. Carol had been hospitalized briefly the previous summer, but she felt that the 40 mg of Prozac on which she had been discharged would help her along. She denied any suicidal ideation at the time of our first session.

At this point, let us consider the information that we have about Carol and how the authorization for 10 sessions may affect our thoughts about treatment. Any therapist, no matter what model of therapy he or she is trained in, must make some choices as to how to best treat such an at-risk patient. This therapist's orientation included the following questions:

How can systems thinking offer greater benefits within a cost-containment framework? What is the context in which the patient's *current* depression is occurring and can that be changed, altered, or supported in some way? Can the efficiency of systems work be maximized further by involving the parents? How can the needs of this depressed individual be addressed and yet be compatible with managed care's maxim of "problem-focused, goal-oriented" therapy so that the *therapy is not compromised*? Is *her* time limit such that we must think about partializing the treatment goals for now so that she may return to college as planned? The Hippocratic oath includes the caution to "do no harm," which for therapists should mean "Do not start something that cannot be finished!" Not a definitive list, but enough of a beginning.

At the end of the first session, this therapist's formulations were as follows:

1. Since Carol was living here, at a distance from family, friends, and in unfamiliar surroundings, treating her in a "vacuum," that is, alone, did not seem therapeutically safe or sound. Further, since Carol indicated that her mother would again want to know what was happening in therapy and her father was portrayed as leaving most of the decisions to his wife, it seemed easier to include both parents in the therapy. Carol was delighted with the thought but was sure that her parents, who lived an hour and a half away, would refuse. When telephoned, although hesitant at first, they agreed to come for the remaining sessions.

2. How could the therapist and the family understand Carol's continuing depression in such a way that some change might be possible in how she was handling her life in order to lower the risk for relapse and still be amenable to the limitations of managed care?

3. Initially each member of the family would need to state and be validated for what he or she thought was the problem. As frequently happens, defining the seriousness of Carol's depression and what should be "done" about it brought out differing ideas of "cause" and course of action between the two parents. Open dialogue between the parents and in front of Carol could begin to interrupt the "collusive" and "intrusive" relationship between mother and daughter, which the two women had previously maintained.

4. As a systems therapist, what could one learn about the circularity of the family's behavioral and verbal interactions that would be clinically useful and expedite the treatment process? If this mother's behavior is viewed as overly attentive reframed from "intrusive" to her daughter's emotional state, what is the reciprocal process in Carol's behavior that keeps this pattern of interaction continuing?

5. A more traditional therapeutic approach might have viewed one

of Carol's problems as "separation–individuation," with mother described as overly close and the father as more distant. As a systems therapist, one finds it more expeditious to strengthen the relationship between the patient and parent who appears less involved, thus rebalancing the system more easily and efficiently.

6. Efforts to "separate" the closer dyad are usually experienced negatively, frequently leading to resistance and/or drop-out from treatment. In any event, it is a far slower and more tedious process to achieve.

7. Finally, since Carol had made it quite clear that she would not quit college, a tentative hypothesis was formulated. A hypothesis must be "systemic," that is, "it must account for all the elements in a problem situation and how they link together" (Boscolo et al., 1987, p. 10). Despite Carol's complaints, being a confidante to her mother marked that relationship as "special" and also probably deflected some of the nagging that would have been directed to the father. His promise to put both children through college even if the family home had to be sold had placed Carol in an untenable position in that at the same time the mother threatened divorce when Carol graduated. Her brother, about to form his own family, had left her "holding the bag," so to speak. For Carol, one way to "prevent" her parents' divorce would be to remain a student forever or to "drop out" of school due to serious depression and/or as a suicide risk. Forming such a hypothesis, if subsequently supported by further data, has nothing to do with the *truth* or the *unconscious* but is useful in formulating an appropriate treatment plan.

At the initial session with the family, everyone was clear about the number of sessions allowed. The parents gave background information about the family, in which Carol had been quite accurate, and were genuinely puzzled about their daughter's intense sadness. As we chatted, the arrangements for the brother's forthcoming wedding were being questioned, which demonstrated each person's difficulties within the family even as they were dealing with this event.

An acrimonious tone had evolved between Carol's family and her brother's in-laws-to-be as mother tried to ensure the necessary social graces for those events she was allowed to plan. Carol was more concerned with the actual ceremony and the bridesmaids' dresses, which had been selected by her brother's fiancée. She felt that the style was designed to make her look even heavier, and invoking her role as the "black sheep," refused to be part of the wedding party. The father tried to remove himself from these discussions, thus infuriating his wife. The brother, who was seen only once, firmly supported the dress selection made by his fiancee and her mother.

Outcome: Following the session with her brother, Carol mailed suicide notes to all family relatives but was "saved" by a fortuitous telephone call as mother later explained it. (No suicide attempt was made.) In fact, at the next session, the family appeared very calm. Carol's explanation was that as the black sheep of the family, she was simply in the way. This therapist responded that rather than "disappearing," she would have been upstaging her brother's wedding by having a funeral first. The effect was profound! For the first time, the father became assertive about what he wanted for his family, with the mother listening. Together the parents discussed how to help Carol find a place within the wedding party, but also, following the therapist's example, held her responsible for her own behavior. Carol's anger toward her brother was seen as isomorphic to that of her parents, which was handled in the remaining sessions. Family-of-origin material concerning the mother/daughter dyad enhanced a shift in Carol's perception of her mother, allowing more open dialogue with her father.

A 6-month follow-up with the family indicated that the wedding had gone well and that everyone had a good time. Likewise, the counselor at college to whom Carol returned for a couple of sessions, reported that although they could not "pinpoint" what had taken place, Carol was happier and for the first time was involving herself in social activities.

The task here has been to demonstrate the effectiveness of family systems therapy within or despite the limitations of managed care. By elaborating our thinking about the information obtained in the first interview and illustrating some of the techniques described earlier, we hope that we have enabled the reader to appreciate the wide range of possibilities which work effectively and efficiently.

MANAGED CARE: COMPATIBLE OR COMBUSTIBLE

In the above section we have tried to show with case examples how family systems therapy can have a reasonable outcome by being problem-focused and effecting behavioral change with a limited number of sessions, compatible with the goals of managed care. Although there will always be valid exceptions to setting "time limits," as with catastrophic illness, for which some insurance must be made available, we believe that regardless of managed care or an indemnity insurance plan, family systems therapy is the most productive, effective, efficient, and respectful way to work with patients who want better lives for themselves and their families.

As we have examined the context in which family therapy developed, an understanding of the emergence of managed care in this country may be helpful.

The American culture, built on the highly regarded "individuality" of each person, continues to focus on the ideal of a white, Anglo-Saxon Protestant, two-parent "happy" patriarchal family and society despite our knowledge and experience to the contrary. The attempts to change the outmoded sexist paradigm of patriarchy has been more successful in the workplace, despite the "glass ceiling," than in the home. For example, despite the statistics on single-headed households, we still cling to the idea that girls and boys can develop "normally" *only* if they each have the same-sex parent for a role model. Given the rate of divorce, usually leading to female-headed households, those attitudes are challenged by Silverstein (Silverstein & Rashbaum, 1995).

Our country holds dear its independent, pioneer spirit (witness the "Marlboro man"), in contrast to our European friends who take pride in their collective histories dating back some two thousand years. Perhaps because we lack such longevity in historical and relational terms, not enough "living" has taken place for us to develop a social conscience. Our health care delivery system is just such an example. Other western industrialized countries have mandated an equitable, single-payor health system for all their citizens, supported by taxes. It would seem that if the profit motive and special-interest groups were not involved, such a plan would surely be on its way here too. The outrage felt by both therapists *and* patients alike has to do with the question of what benefits (read entitlements) we should have but for which this country is unwilling to pay even as the demand for tax cuts continues.

From this mentality arise escalating health costs *and* a "cut-the-fat mentality," which has produced, some might say, the pork barrel of managed care. That managed care seeks to have the most effective, least restrictive, high-quality medicine is laudable; the fact that it is governed by insurance companies who are in the business of making a profit is contradictory.

Past consumer experience has been rooted in traditional indemnity coverage, a luxury that we can no longer afford. A recent study of utilization patterns for outpatient psychotherapy found that "long-term psychotherapy (over twenty visits) accounted for 15.7% of psychotherapy users and 62.9% of total psychotherapy expenditures" (Olfson & Fincus, 1994, p. 1289). We need to realize that while managed care is not necessarily a done deal, some form of *health care rationing for this country is here to stay*. Of course, "health care—and everything else in American life—has always been 'rationed' to the poor, but this is the first time that masses of middle-class Americans will experience the limitations" (Wylie, 1994) of benefits to which they think they are "entitled."

Perhaps because some forms of limited benefits have come later to the psychiatric community, we have been caught off guard. For example when Congress in 1982 astonished the medical world by using the formula of diagnosis related groups (DRGs) to *limit* the benefits of the Medicare-Medicaid populations on inpatient length of stay (LOS), English and his colleagues, in their much heralded APA study, found compelling evidence for exemption of DRG regulation for inpatient psychiatry (English et al., 1986).

Another study (Mezzich & Coffman, 1985, p. 1262) found a "patient's symptomatology, level of adaptive functioning, and social supports" to be more important predictors of LOS than diagnosis for psychiatric usage, and we believe the same holds true for outpatient therapy as well. Those attributes are certainly at the top of the agenda for managed care, but with inherent difficulties: (1) the number of sessions allowed which managed care correlates with diagnosis, (2) the requirement for a DSM-IV (A.P.A., 1994) *individual* diagnostic code for reimbursement, and all of which are discussed later in this chapter, and (3) the requirement for an Axis I diagnosis to justify continuing treatment.

Nevertheless, there are many compatibilities between family systems therapy and managed care companies, even though they have emerged from different points of view. Managed care requires working within a specific time frame, setting manageable goals, and demonstrating evidence of behavioral goals. The training of marriage and family therapists (MFTs), with perhaps the exception of the object-relations school, focuses on just such criteria: attention to behavioral patterns and interactions that influence (emotional) functioning and helping the patient within the least amount of time, thereby "banking" unused sessions in case of future need. Marriage and family therapists move treatment away from "pathologizing" past relationships or victimization by an emphasis on empowerment and using patients own resources—just what the managed care companies say they want. Our approach in defining the problem with the patient(s), discussed earlier, does just that. With their clients, MFTs cocreate a context saying that what happens outside the therapy room (least restrictive environment) is more important than what happens inside (Tilley, 1993, p. 12).

In fact, as family systems therapists, if we look at the demise of reimbursable open-ended ego-reconstructive psychotherapies and the reaction that many therapists are experiencing, we might also wonder about the reciprocal process for those they treat who may have become all too comfortable with their "patienthood."

At the same time, however, this therapist has noticed a greater variety of people who are now seeking help. One reason may be that these newer patients, who have not been "trained" in long-term therapy, are quite content with a limited time frame and number of sessions. Rather than experiencing these elements as a deterrent, they are seeking help to solve a particular problem without the fear of being seduced into treatment with no end, an unfortunate reputation of psychotherapy. A study of time-limited psychotherapy supports this thesis in demonstrating that "the dropout rate for patients in brief psychotherapy in which the length of therapy was specified at the outset of treatment ... was about one-half the dropout rate for patients in brief but unspecified time limit and long-term therapy" (Sledge et al., 1990, p. 1341). One might even venture to say that managed care companies are trying to validate the good use of therapy.

This therapist has observed that frequently length of treatment or number of sessions requested by the therapist is a function of how a problem is defined. A systems approach is mindful of the *context* in which the therapy is taking place, so that a shared perception between patient and therapist of what "works well" and "what needs changing" can be developed, which then helps formulate the task at hand and the direction the therapy should take. Together we discuss number of sessions allowed, how best to use the time effectively, and how this therapist will handle outpatient treatment reports (OTRs) and possible requests for more sessions. These criteria rarely become issues in and of themselves unless there is a "need" for the patient *or* therapist to triangulate some (one) thing into the therapy. If the therapy has reached an impasse or the issues being dealt with are too anxiety-provoking, blame can always be "projected" onto another person (a grandparent), or object (the bottle) to relieve the tension—or in this case the managed care companies. Yet that is what systems work is all about, calling for a profound understanding of context (managed care) and how individuals, couples, families, and therapists can function within its limitations.

It is unfortunate, therefore, that managed care companies retain such a rigid concept from the traditional psychiatric paradigm in equating number of sessions to number of weeks. Well known in systems work is that the "number of hours with a family is small but the length of time needed for family reorganization can be very long" (Hoffman, 1981, p. 287). This concept has proven effective, as demonstrated by Selvini-Palazzoli and her colleagues in Milan, particularly in their work with disorganized families whose appointments might be scheduled between two weeks and several months apart (Selvini-Palazzoli, 1978). Understandably, it becomes burdensome for family systems therapists to have to submit the required additional paperwork or clinical telephone review for a time extension even though no additional sessions are needed or requested.

Nevertheless, where family systems therapy and the managed care professional ethos part company is in the latter's total reliance on the medical model diagnosis as a determinant for number of sessions needed for appropriate treatment. "Our whole diagnostic system is geared to measuring illness, not health or how well somebody functions" (Bower, in Wylie, 1994).

Further, this approach negates the usefulness of the biopsychosocial model, which informs us about human functioning on many levels. The importance of any scientific model "is measured not by whether it is right or wrong but by how useful it is" (Engel, 1980, p. 543).

In this regard, the more traditional stance of describing patients in DSM-IV with pathologic characteristics that reside *within* a patient is a diagnostic "stance that runs directly counter to systemic or other formulations of client difficulties as perceived by family therapists" (Strong, 1993, p. 251). Furthermore, it tells the clinician very little of *what* to do in treatment planning. For example, if the therapist had believed that Hedda's daughter Nellie (case example, page 126), had "internalized" her mother's image or was acting out the "repetition compulsion syndrome," it would have continued the negative concept the mother already held about herself.

Because conceptualizing a patient's difficulty in this way limits *thinking* about possible solutions or creative alternatives, interest in the relational diagnoses has developed as clinicians have "come to believe that many disorders emanate from interpersonal problems rather than from intrapsychic distress" (Kaslow, 1993, p. 255).

For example, we believe the "success" in helping the White family (case example, page 125) had to do with conceptualizing the family arguments as a reciprocal process, which then produced each individual's own idiosyncratic way of responding to a situation in order to address the serious and recurrent difficulties between family members, no doubt influenced by the father's intermittent alcoholism (addressed during the course of treatment). Focusing on each individual's responsibility for behavior within the context of the family allowed a profound change in family functioning in a relatively short time; what managed care companies say they want. By contrast, restructuring the father's character pathology with a viable DSM-IV diagnosis while trying to meet the criteria for "medical necessity" is a long-term proposition for which managed care would not have paid, nor would it have helped this family enjoy a pleasant celebration.

We do not know about "long-term" outcome with this family, nor should that even be a criterion for "success." What is very important is that the family experienced a different way of behaving, which then opens the possibility of *choice* about future behavior together.

Even with major illnesses such as schizophrenia and bipolar disorders which research suggests a biological basis of the diseases, numerous studies (Vaughn & Leff, 1976; Anderson, Hogarty, & Reiss, 1980; Falloon & Liberman, 1983; Hogarty et al., 1986; McFarlane et al., 1995) have shown that family relationships, social context, and community resources can influence the *course* of the illness. This should be of major interest to the managed care companies, because when these patients relapse, rehospitalization is frequently necessary—an expensive proposition. By contrast, patients in other diagnostic categories who regress can usually continue treatment as outpatients. Since psychoeducation is not listed in the DSM-IV because it is not an illness, reimbursement can only be achieved by slightly unethical means, listing another family member, usually the mother, with a "suitable" diagnosis.

What we are suggesting here is that a multiaxial view as a criterion for diagnostic purposes is more useful, more relevant, and more economical for helping patients. In noting that "a defect of the current diagnostic manual is the explicit restriction to syndromes that occur 'in a person,' " the Group for the Advancement of Psychiatry (GAP) Committee on the Family were concerned that V codes which are vague and nonreimbursable do not denote the seriousness of a relational situation—for example, incest—nor the burden placed on families with severely and persistently mentally ill relatives as detailed above. They recommended "recognition of syndromes that are best defined and identified as occurring between persons, as relational or interpersonal syndromes . . . (which) often entail serious personal dysfunction and warrant inclusion as mental disorders" (Group for the Advancement of Psychiatry Committee on the Family, 1989, p. 1492).

In addition to Axis I clarification, we regard Axis IV, the rating scale indicating severity of psychosocial stressors, acute events, and/or enduring circumstances critical for treatment planning. Every example of stressors in the DSM-III-R (1987) mentions *another* (person or circumstance) involved with the primary patient; DSM-IV goes further in recognizing difficulties in various groups with *others*. These are not intrapsychic phenomena. Since Axis IV shows some understanding about the *context* in which a patient seeks psychiatric help (except self-enlightenment), it is most curious that these events are abandoned to intrapsychic phenomena by therapists when formulating treatment and frequently ignored by the managed care companies.

Perhaps Axis V is where the greatest divergence occurs between the individually oriented therapists and those of us in the family field. While Goldman and colleagues are correct in noting that Axis V, Global Assessment of Functioning Scale, as a single axis used for the combination of psychological, social, and occupational functioning "violates the principal of a multiaxial system (Goldman et al., 1992, p. 1151), their modification is nevertheless individually based. A subsequent field trial (Patterson & Lee, 1995) supports this modification by using the Social and Occupational Functioning Assessment Scale (SOFAS) now included in DSM-IV (A.P.A., p. 761).

To our way of thinking, this is insufficient to obtain the information needed for good treatment planning. Since 1975, the efforts of Lyman Wynne, a highly regarded psychiatrist, have continuously stressed an understanding of a biopsychosocial context, which inherently includes relationships. A modest acceptance of this thinking has been the inclusion of the Global Assessment of Relational Functioning Scale (GARF) in the DSM-IV (A.P.A. pp. 758–759). With the publication of the "Handbook of Relational Diagnosis (1996), the stage may just be set for "a philosophic shift to a systemic framework" (Kaslow, 1993, p. 259).

How can the information outlined above be useful for preventative action and as a focus for the direction of treatment planning? How can this new information affect managed care decisions? If we recall the case of Carol (case example, p. 129), the therapist elected not to treat her major depression as an intrapsychic illness but worked with the family to shift the balance of their relationships, which not only alleviated the depression but also constructed a safety net for their daughter.

By contrast, a managed care company, who had already sent a directive to providers stating that in their desire for "quality" and "efficacy" they wished to utilize a 10-session model for diseases including major depression, referred just such a patient.

> Vera, a white woman in her mid-forties, requested help in ending a long-standing relationship with a married man. She herself was divorced for almost a year but allowed her ex-husband to continue living with her out of fear of being alone. She had recently purchased a condominium and although she had moved in, was feeling lonely and depressed: her fantasy that she could spend more time with the boyfriend never materialized. She cried frequently at work. Although not on good terms with her mother, who lived in the area, Vera nevertheless asked her to sleep over occasionally because she was frightened to be alone. Her only girlfriend kept in regular contact. On initial contact, a Thursday, this therapist was impressed by Vera's profound depression and the absence of any meaningful, stable relationship in her life. Hospitalization was recommended without a psychiatric evaluation because the managed care's local psychiatrist could not offer an appointment until the following Tuesday. Except for her mother, this therapist maintained telephone contact with all the above and the local Crisis Team until Vera was admitted on Monday morning.

The next this therapist heard about Vera was a month later, when I telephoned her friend. A well-known psychiatric hospital had admitted Vera for 2 weeks (without contacting this therapist) and then discharged her to her mother's home, with a therapy appointment later in the week. Vera went out the window to her death the next day.

The stupidity, greed, or ignorance of the managed care company and the hospital's stupidity or greed (a discounted managed care fee?) or feigned ignorance of successful discharge procedures (Altman, 1983) hastened the demise of this patient.

Both Carol and Vera had the same diagnoses: Axis I, Major Depressive Episode, recurrent; Axis IV moderate (Carol, chronic parental discord and Vera, marital separation); Axis V is in the 41–50 category.

Nevertheless, the ability of the one depressed patient to continue functioning despite her illness and suicide threat while the other patient gave up altogether should raise an alarm as to our basic beliefs about criteria in these diagnostic categories and how they are used by therapists and managed care alike. The risk factors for Vera were very clear yet not clearly documentable on the existing Axis V. If the GARF in DSM-IV were to receive legitimate acceptance as a rating scale, one would find that Vera's score would read "Relational unit is obviously and seriously dysfunctional; forms and time periods of satisfactory relating are rare" (DSM-IV, p. 759). By contrast, Carol's score, one category higher, would read, "Relational unit has occasional times of satisfying and competent functioning together, but clearly dysfunctional, unsatisfying relationships tend to predominate (DSM-IV, p. 759). If this rating scale were to be acknowledged by the psychiatric establishment it could denote the severity of illness more reliably thus affording greater specificity in treatment planning.

If we consider it essential that managed care take a broader perspective in its view of patient functioning what should be said about the training of those who choose to work within the managed care paradigm? Some suggest "retraining" master's level clinicians, the largest provider category (and the poorest-paid), "since social workers and psychiatric nurses have often been trained only in long-term psychotherapy approaches" (Patterson & Berman, 1991, p. 28).

Jay Haley astutely and irreverently points out "how few meetings and training programs there are on how to do long-term therapy. . . . The implication is that everyone knows how to engage clients in therapy for years. Yet long-term therapists are made, not born. Therapists do not have innate skills in committing clients to long-term contracts. Without training, they must learn by trial and error to do interminable therapy when they get into practice" (Haley, 1990, p. 32).

At the other end of the spectrum, a national conference forum is offering a 1-day seminar in brief strategic therapy promising that clinicians "will learn how to implement short-term strategic interventions for problems of self-esteem, anxiety, attention deficits, conduct disorders and dysfunctional family relationships" (Benson, 1995, p. 22). All in 1 day! We believe this might meet the criterion for the true definition of "band-aid" therapy.

CONCLUSION

Throughout this chapter, it has been documented that by training, family systems therapists are prepared for what I believe to be the most effective, efficient, and respectful therapy for the coming years. That this training turns out to be compatible with many of managed care's goals is initially coincidental. This compatibility may be fortuitous, however, for the many patients who are enrolled in some form of managed health plan.

The case examples may give the reader, more experienced in traditional therapy practice, inspiration to learn about this work, which is as practical as it is creative.

Finally, what is considered to be some of the most serious deficiencies in our profession, as well as the criteria used by managed care, have been addressed in the last section. The continuing adherence to the "way it used to be", as well as a resistance to validate newer findings in human relationships and mental illness as criteria for the practice of psychotherapy, seems counterproductive. Is it so difficult for our profession to adapt to change; that which we profess we are helping our patients to do?

REFERENCES

Ackerman Institute for Family Therapy: *Current*. New York: Ackerman Institute.
Ackerman, N. W. (1937). The family as a social and emotional unit. In D. Bloch & R. Simon (eds.) (1982). *The strength of family therapy* (pp. 153–158). New York: Brunner/Mazel.
Alperin, R. M. (1994). Managed care versus psychoanalytic psychotherapy: Conflicting ideologies. *Clinical Social Work Journal*, 22(2), 137–148.
Altman, H. (1995). A response to Richard Alperin's article "Managed care versus psychoanalytic psychotherapy: Conflicting ideologies. *Clinical Social Work Journal*, 23, 223–226.
Altman, H. (1983). A collaborative approach to discharge planning for chronic mental patients. *Hospital and Community Psychiatry*, 34, 641–642.
Altman-Jacobs, H. (1958). The week-end visits at home. A study of family members relationships and roles during the hospitalized child's visit at home. Masters thesis, Simmons College School of Social Work.
American Psychiatric Association (3rd ed. revised, Washington, D.C.: American Psychiatric Association.

American Psychiatric Association (1994). Diagnostic and statistical manual of mental disorders (4th ed.). Washington, DC.

Anderson, C. M., Hogarty, G. E., and Reiss, D. J. (1980). Family treatment of adult schizophrenic patients: a psycho-educational approach. Schizophrenia Bulletin, 6, 490–505.

Aponte, H. J., & Van Deusen, J. M. (1981). Structural family therapy. In A. S. Gurman (ed.) *Handbook of family therapy* (pp. 310–360). New York: Brunner/Mazel.

Benson, G. L., (1995). *Brief strategic therapy with children, adolescents and parents*. American Health Care Institute.

Boscolo, L., Gianfranco, C., Hoffman, L., & Penn, P. (1987). *Milan systemic family therapy: Conversations in theory and practice*. New York: Basic Books.

Bowen, M. (1976). Theory in the practice of psychotherapy. In P. J. Guerin (Ed.). *Family therapy theory and practice* (pp. 42–90). New York: Gardner Press.

Bower, M. In Wylie, M. (1994). Endangered species. *The Family Therapy Networker, 18*, 20–33.

Engel, G. L. (1980). The clinical application of the biopsychosocial model. *American Journal Psychiatry, 137*, 535–544.

English, J. T., Sharfstein, S. S., Scherl, D. J., et al. (1986). Diagnosis-related groups and general hospital psychiatry: The APA study. *American Journal of Psychiatry, 143*, 131–139.

Erickson, M. H. (1974). *Change: Principles of problem formation and problem resolution*. New York: W. W. Norton.

Falloon, I. R. H., & Liberman, R. P. (1983). Behavioral family interventions in the management of chronic schizophrenia. In W. R. McFarlane (Ed.). *Family Therapy in Schizophrenia* (pp. 117–137). New York: Guilford Press.

Frances, A., Clarkin, J. F., & Perry, S. (1984). DSM-III and family therapy. *American Journal of J Psychiatry, 141*, 406.

Goldberg, J. R. (1993). MFTs, others push for relational diagnosis. *Family Therapy News, 24*, p. 19.

Goldman, H. H., Skodol, A. E., & Lave, T. R. (1992). Revising Axis V for DSM-IV: A review of measures of social functioning. *American Journal of Psychiatry, 149*, 1148–1156.

Group for the Advancement of Psychiatry Committee on the Family. (1989). The challenge of relational diagnoses: Applying the biopsychosocial model in DSM-IV. *American Journal of Psychiatry, 146*, 1492–1494.

Guerin, P. J. (1976). *Family therapy theory and practice*. New York: Gardner Press.

Gurman, A. S., & Kniskern, D. P. (1981). *Handbook of family therapy*. New York: Brunner/Mazel.

Haley, J. (1990). Interminable therapy. *The Family Therapy Networker, 14*, 32.

Haley, J. (1989). *Problem-solving therapy*, San Francisco: Jossey-Bass.

Hoffman, L. (1981). *Foundations in family therapy*. New York: Basic Books.

Hogarty, G. E., Anderson, C. M., Reiss, D. J., et al. (1986). Family psychoeducation, social skills training, and maintenance chemotherapy in the aftercare treatment of schizophrenia. *Archives of General Psychiatry, 43*, 633–642.

Journal of Marital and Family Therapy: (Special Edition) 1995, *21* (4) pp. 339–623.

Karls, J. M. Wandrei, K. E. (1992). PIE: A new language for social work. *Social Work, 37*, p. 80.

Kaslow, F. W. (1993). Relational diagnosis: An idea whose time has come. *Family Process, 32*, 255–259.

Kaslow, F. W. (1966). *Handbook of Relational Diagnosis and Dysfunctional Family Patterns.* New York: John Wiley.

Kerr, M. E. (1981). Family systems theory and therapy. In A. S. Gurman & D. P. Kniskern (Eds.). *Handbook of family therapy* (pp. 226–264). New York: Brunner/Mazel.

Marmor, J. (1983). Systems thinking in psychiatry: Some theoretical and clinical implications. *American Journal of Psychiatry. 140*, 833–838.

McFarlane, W. R., Link, B., Dushay, R., et al. (1995). Psychoeducational multiple family groups: Four-year relapse outcome in schizophrenia. *Family Process, 34*, 127–144.

Mezzich, J. E., & Coffman, G. A. (1985). Factors influencing length of hospital stay. *Hospital and Community Psychiatry, 36*, 1262–1270.

Minuchin, S., Montalvo, B., Guerney, et al. (1967). *Families of the slums.* New York: Basic Books.

Olfson, M., Pincus, H. A. (1994). Outpatient psychotherapy in the United States: II. Patterns of utilization. *American Journal of Psychiatry, 151*, 1289.

Papp, P. (1983). *The process of change.* New York: Guilford Press.

Patterson, D. Y., & Berman, W. H. (1991). Organizational and service delivery issues in managed mental health services. In C. S. Austad & W. H. Berman, (Eds.). Psychotherapy in managed health care. Washington, DC: American Psychological Association.

Patterson, D. A., & Lee, M. S., (1995). Field trial of the global assessment of functioning scale-modified. *American Journal of Psychiatry. 152*:1386–1388.

Riché-Ault, M., (1983). Integrating families into a healing community: The use of structural and strategic family therapy in a psychodynamically-oriented hospital. *Residental Group Care & Treatment. 1*(4), 67–83.

Selvini-Palazzoli, M. (1978). *Paradox & counterparadox: A new model on the treatment of the family in schizophrenic transaction.* Northvale, NJ: Jason Aronson.

Selvini-Palazzoli, M., Boscolo, L., Cecchin, G., & Prata, G. (1980). Hypothesizing-circularity-neutrality: Three guidelines for the conductor of the session. *Family Process, 19*, 3–12.

Silverstein, O. (1987). The application of family therapy skills in work with individuals (unpublished manuscript).

Silverstein, O., & Rashbaum, B. (1995). *The courage to raise good men.* New York: Penguin Books.

Simmons, D. S., Doherty, W. J. (1995). Defining who we are and what we do: clinical practice patterns of marriage and family therapists in Minnesota. Journal of Marital and Family Therapy. *21* 3–16.

Simon, R. (1984a). Stranger in a strange land. *The Family Therapy Networker, 8*, 21–25.

Simon, R., (1984b). From ideology to practice. *The Family Therapy Networker*. 8(3), 28–40.

Sledge, W. H., Moras, K., Hartley, D., & Levine, M. (1990). Effect of time-limited psychotherapy on patient dropout rates. *American Journal of Psychiatry, 147*, 1341–1347.

Sprenkle, D. H. and Bailey, C. E. (1995). Editor's Introduction, Journal of Marital and Family Therapy, *21*, 339–340.

Strong, T. (1993). Commentary: DSM-IV and describing problems in family therapy. *Family Process, 32*, 249–253.

Terkelsen, K. G. (1983). A schizophrenia and the family: II. Adverse effects of family therapy. Family Process, 22, 191–200.

Tilley, K. A. (1993). Making the cut: Family therapists and managed care. *Family Therapy News, 24*, 12–13.

Vaughn, C. E., & Leff, J. P. (1976). The influence of family and social factors on the course of psychiatric illness: A comparison of schizophrenic and depressed neurotic patients. *British Journal of Psychiatry, 129*, 125–137.

Walters, M., Carter, B., Papp, P., & Silverstein, O. (1988). *The invisible web: Gender patterns in family relationships*. New York: Guilford Press.

Watzlawick, P., Weakland, J., & Fisch, R. (1974). *Change*: Principles of problem formation and problem resolution. New York: W. W. Norton.

Weakland, J. In Wylie, M. (1990). Brief therapy on the couch. *The Family Therapy Networker, 14*, 26–35.

Williams, J. B. W., Goldman, H. H., Gruenberg, A., et al. (1990). The multiaxial system. *Hospital and Community Psychiatry. 41*, 1181–1182.

Williams, J. B. W., Karls, J. M., & Wandrei, K. E., (1989). The-person-in-environment (PIE) system for describing problems of social functioning. *Hospital & Community Psychiatry, 40*, 1125–1127.

Wylie, M. (1994). Endangered species. *The Family Therapy Networker. 18*, 20–33.

CHAPTER 8

Hypnotherapy and Managed Care

William Ballen
Kent Jarratt

Managed care evolved within the context of short-term treatment. Because hypnosis is a short-term treatment, it should flourish in the managed care environment. However, to date this has not been the case. There has been no widespread acceptance of hypnosis by managed care. Rather, treatments under the catchall phrase *cognitive-behavior* have taken precedence, particularly as therapists and agencies scramble to find the right words that will be acceptable to provider relations personnel and peer review managers. We feel that hypnosis has been underutilized primarily because of myths about hypnosis and outdated definitions. Although hypnosis has been designated as an approved medical procedure by the American Medical Association since 1954, there is still a great deal of misunderstanding about it, especially within the community of managed care providers responsible for the delivery of mental health services, who are often not aware of recent research. Yet, there has been an explosion of research in the use of hypnosis in psychophysiologic disorders such as asthma, skin diseases, gastrointestinal disorders, pain, and immune-related diseases. The hypnotic treatment of habit disorders such as smoking, overeating, substance abuse and alcoholism, sexual dysfunctions, and sleep disturbances is also on the rise (Brown & Fromm, 1986). Still, many managed care companies are either unwilling to authorize hypnotic treatment or will authorize treatment only if a psychiatrist is consulted first. Frequently, the managed care psychiatrist is not an expert in hypnosis and most likely has no knowledge of its clinical use other than knowing from history books that Freud once employed it as an abreactive technique and then stopped using it. Too often, unfortunately, this has been the lens through which managed care views hypnosis.

The purpose of this chapter is to show that hypnosis can claim a unique position within short-term treatment models and that it should be able to take root in a managed care environment. As we define hypnosis and illustrate its particular uses, we will focus on which patients are appropriate for this treatment as well as which patients are not, discuss treatment goals within a managed care context, look at the limitations of managed care, and discuss how these limitations can be addressed and resolved. It is our hope that by placing hypnosis and hypnotherapy within its historical context as a short-term treatment modality, managed care will increasingly see hypnosis and hypnotherapy not only as relevant and justifiable but as a treatment of choice for a substantial number of patients.

DISPELLING THE MYTHS—HISTORICAL PERSPECTIVE

Managed care is not unique as an institution in needing to be updated on the uses and effectiveness of hypnosis. Except within a circumscribed community of therapists, hypnosis is underutilized in the mental health field as a whole. It is important, then, that a workable model of hypnosis be presented so that myths, some of which are propagated within our own field, can be dispelled. A workable model of hypnosis must seek answers to two types of questions: What is hypnosis and what is it not. Over the past hundred years, since Freud's early writings on hypnosis, and to this day, there has been a tendency in the literature to equate hypnosis only with suggestibility. In fact, Bernheim, who after Charcot became Freud's foremost mentor in hypnosis, equated hypnosis mechanistically with a state of suggestibility. As we will see, this view of hypnosis, despite its subsequent clinical and experimental invalidation, persists today. It is perhaps this viewpoint, with its exclusive emphasis on the hypnotist as an all-powerful figure who plants suggestions in the patient, that understandably makes managed care consultants hesitant to approve treatment.

It was, indeed, Freud's initial belief in the power of hypnotic suggestion that led him to think that he could remove hysterical symptoms by simple abreaction and suggestion. When this proved futile, Freud wrote: "I gave up the suggestion technique, and with it hypnosis, so early in my practice because I despaired of making suggestion powerful and enduring enough to effect permanent cures" (Kline, 1954).

The scientific investigation of hypnosis has advanced considerably since

Freud's time. However, due to Freud's unrivaled position in the history of psychoanalysis, most psychoanalysts and psychotherapists working within the psychoanalytic model know less about hypnosis today than Freud did in 1885. Is this what Freud the scientist would have wanted? It is doubtful, for he was impressed with the effectiveness of hypnosis in dealing with war neuroses and the trauma of combat and wrote that it might be necessary to again consider the value of hypnosis in psychotherapy. At the end of his life, in 1939, he wrote the following:

> There are many ways and means of practicing psychotherapy. All that lead to recovery are good. We have developed the technique of hypnotic suggestion, and psychotherapy. . . . I despise none of these methods and would use them all under the proper conditions. If I have actually come to confine myself to one form of treatment . . . it is because I have allowed myself to be influenced by purely subjective motives [Kline, 1954].

DEFINING HYPNOSIS

As already mentioned, one reason why hypnosis is underutilized by managed care is because a clear, operational definition of hypnosis is often lacking. What is it, exactly, that a hypnotherapist does to a patient, and how does the patient experience this interaction? Therefore, any discussion of the use of hypnosis within a managed care environment must begin with an expanded definition of hypnosis that draws from current research.

At one time, it was erroneously believed that in hypnosis the subject's ego was bypassed; that he was so regressed that he gave over his ego and superego functioning to the person of the hypnotherapist. Today we know that the subject's ego and its defenses are very much involved in hypnosis, albeit differently than in a waking state. It may be that it is precisely the increased activity and receptivity of the ego to stimuli from without and within in hypnosis that is at the heart of a contemporary understanding of the therapeutic action of hypnotherapy. People in hypnosis maintain the capacity to observe, reflect, monitor, and direct their experiences if they choose to. Just as people cannot be hypnotized against their wills or made to carry out behaviors that are antagonistic to their own values and self-interests, people have greater access to ego functions in hypnosis and can move with greater facility back and forth between bipolar aspects of the ego. There is enhanced affective responsiveness and imagery production in hypnosis as well as the ability to dissociate affect from cognition and the reverse. The concentrated attention and absorption can, in a moment, become diffuse, allowing for a psychic mobility that enables movement between different or even opposite states. The ability to vacillate between conscious and unconscious, past and present, between ego-activity and ego-receptivity, observation and experience, between enhanced memory and amnesia, or mind and body is the *sine qua non* of hypnotherapy. This flexibility, inherent in hypnotherapy is what often makes it so effective in unblocking stalled treatments. It is this characteristic fluidity that constitutes its distinct advantage over waking-state therapy (Fromm, in Fromm & Nash, 1992).

The hypnotist does not control the patient's consciousness or state of consciousness but rather helps the patient to access a natural ability to move from one state to the other. The hypnotist leads the patient to "discover" her trance state and to utilize it. Some patients are more naturally skilled at doing this while others need more direction from the hypnotist.

Here is an elegant definition of hypnosis that speaks to its potential for managed care: "In many ways hypnosis is the art of securing a patient's attention and then effectively communicating ideas that enhance motivation and change perceptions" (Hammond, 1990).

Central to any process of psychotherapeutic change is the alteration of the individual's perception of self, his or her world, and the relation between the two. For there to be perception, there must be a sensory apparatus. Visual, auditory, somatosensory, auditory, and gustatory mechanisms, along with a sense of time, are the means by which we take in information—about the world outside as well as inside ourselves. Without the ability to sense or perceive data from within and without or where the perception is flawed, it becomes difficult to function.

Managed care's emphasis is on short-term treatment models that can most clearly document how and when the patient's altered perception occurs. Because of a need to succinctly document these goals and changes, managed care favors models that can, for example, operate within a particular type of documentation, like the "S.O.A.P." note (Subjective/Objective/Assessment/Plan). These models are favored over more traditional psychoanalytic/psychodynamic models that see changes of perception occurring through the medium of the therapeutic relationship and so, by necessity, chart progress over a vastly expanded time frame. They document this progress in language that is process-oriented rather than goal-directed. With regard to these two trends, where does hypnosis fit? In fact, hypnosis in its current, post-Freudian development has the potential to bridge the process orientation of psychoanalysis with the outcome orientation required of managed care. To begin to develop this link, it is important to answer the question: What constitutes the state of being hypnotized?

THE HYPNOTIC STATE

Hypnosis is an altered state of consciousness characterized by cognitive, perceptual, and psychophysical alterations not present in the waking state (Brown & Fromm, 1986). Cognitive changes involve alterations of attention that can be highly focused on internal or external stimuli. There is heightened absorption and, in deeper states, a shift to primary-process thought. Sensory-perceptual changes often include visual-spatial, somatic-kinesthetic, and auditory-sensory modalities. Psychophysiologic alterations that have been noted in therapeutic hypnosis are reduced respiration and heart rate, with lowered blood pressure and a shift to parasympathetic and right hemispheric functioning. As previously noted, there is, even in light hypnosis, a heightened facility in shifting between observing and experiencing ego and between conscious and unconscious processes.

The hypnotic state is characterized by various phenomena. Recognition and understanding of these phenomena enable the hypnotherapist to utilize them therapeutically. An excellent summary of hypnotic phenomena is presented in *Hypnotherapy and Hypnoanalysis* (Brown & Fromm, 1986); the following section is partially adapted from their book. Specific examples of the utilization of these phenomena are given later in this chapter during our discussion of the types of patients that are appropriate for hypnosis within a managed care context.

YIELDING OF THE GENERALIZED
REALITY ORIENTATION

One of the hallmarks of the hypnotic state is the loosening of the generalized reality orientation. Hypnotic subjects may report feeling detached from their environment. Loud noises and visual stimuli may register with them, but they are rarely distracted or even interested in that which is not relevant to their trance experiences. In deep hypnosis, subjects are so engrossed and absorbed in their own internal processes that they become removed from what goes on around them. There is an inhibition of higher cognitive evaluation of sensory processes. This is seen clearly in the negative and positive hallucinations of subjects in experimental situations (suggested hallucinations are rarely utilized in clinical settings). In positive hallucination, the subject projects on internal visual image into the external world. He sees something that is not there. In reality, for instance, a hallucinated cat may be seen sitting on a chair. Subjects who are genuinely hallucinating are more consistent in their reports of hallucinated phenomena than people in a normal waking state or nonhypnotizable people who are instructed to simulate hypnosis and positive hallucinations. For example, the genuinely hallucinating subjects see the seat of the hallucinated chair through the body of the hallucinated cat on top of it. Genuine hallucinating subjects also shy away from sitting on the chair or will try to shoo away the imagined cat before sitting down. Simulators will just sit down. The same inhibitory mechanism that brings about positive hallucinations also brings out negative hallucinations. Hypnotic deafness is an often quoted example of a negative hallucination, where the hypnotized person does not consciously hear real sounds. There is a similarity between hypnotic deafness and hypnotic anesthesia. In both, although the subjects do not consciously experience the sensory stimuli of sound or induced pain, the recognition of the sensory information can be accessed unconsciously. Hilgard interprets these results as an inhibition of the cognitive reality-oriented appraisal mechanisms by which sensory data are interpreted in the waking state. Hypnotically deaf subjects will not consciously or pre-consciously hear a tone but will react with increased muscle potentials; organically deaf patients will not. Subjects in pain studies will report no pain when given a stimulus that would cause pain in the waking state, yet, if asked, they admit to knowing that they are in pain but say that they just do not feel it. This phenomenon is closely related to what has been termed trance logic or tolerance for incongruity. Trance logic is defined as "the ability of the subject to mix freely his perceptions derived from reality with those that stem from his imagination and are perceived as hallucinations. These perceptions are fused in a manner that ignores everyday logic." Due to the altered information processing in hypnosis, the subject is not bothered by contradictory perceptions or logically inconsistent ideas.

PERCEIVED INVOLUNTARISM

It is important that, in working with a hypnotist, both managed care staff and their patients understand the answers to questions like: Who is really in control? Have they entered into a Svengali-like relationship? As we shall see, the very answer can change the patient's perception of her own mastery.

During hypnosis, many subjects are able to experience ideomotor phenomena. A very common ideomotor phenomenon is arm levitation. Although the subject may subjectively experience his arm lifting up without conscious effort, it is, of course, his capacity for focused attention and imaginative involvement that enables it to move. What the subject in hypnosis may experience as involuntary is nevertheless still under his own goal-directed control. Pointing this out to patients (rather than the therapist exploiting it for his own narcissistic needs) can be quite empowering for the patient. For most hypnotherapy, a good rule of thumb is to credit the patient with the production of all hypnotic phenomena. Patients will often feel a renewed sense of hope and a conviction that they can do things they did not think they could do. With the proper handling, the patient's initial successes in producing and experiencing his own hypnotic abilities are re-framed into ego-building experiences. The experience of something new in hypnosis—the initial interesting change from perceived voluntariness to perceived involuntariness—can give the patient an embryonic sense that change might come more easily to him than his habitual cognitive evalua-tions may have considered. A simple arm levitation or relaxation response during the initial hypnosis, if it is explained as the patient's achievement, will further his sense of efficacy and set a tone for additional positively an-ticipated therapeutic changes in the areas where they are needed. Imagine the reaction of a patient who is led to wonder what other problems he may be able to let go of just as he so quickly learned to let go of all sensation in his arm.

TIME DISTORTION

As with all hypnotic phenomena, time distortion occurs to some degree in everyday waking activity. We have all had the subjective experience of time moving either fast or slowly and thereby overestimating and underestimat-ing the objective time that has elapsed. Usually we experience time as pro-ceeding quickly when an activity is pleasurable and slowly when the activity is not pleasurable (the adage "Time flies when you are having fun" truly reflects a hypnotic phenomenon). Once again, trance serves to augment a mechanism that takes place naturally. Einstein recognized that there is frequently a discrepancy between solar time and what he called "I" time or the more personal subjective experience of time. Because time can be highly condensed or expanded in hypnotic trance, a number of therapeutic applications have been discovered; we review these below. Time distortion can be used with most subjects who develop a moderately deep trance. The subject can be given instructions to complete a task during hypno-sis or later, posthypnotically; although the activity seems to proceed at the normal rate to the subject, it actually takes place with great rapidity. Some of the most dramatic results in the experimental studies of time distortion have come from counting experiments. Cooper and Erickson have reported the following example. (The letter *E* stands for *experimenter*; *S* stands for *subject*.)

E: You're back on the farm, and are going to churn some butter. Tell me what you see.

S: (Subject described the scene in some detail. She was sitting on the back porch with a crockery churn half full of milk. She mentioned the paddle with the "crosspiece" on it, and the hole in the top of the churn, through which the paddle passes.)

E: Now just stay there for a while, and listen carefully. You're going to churn that milk, and it's going to take you ten minutes, which will be plenty of time. While churning, you're going to count the strokes. I shall give you a signal to start, and another signal, at the end of ten minutes, to stop. Here comes the signal— "Start."

                    (three seconds later)

E: Now stop. The ten minutes are up. Now make your mind a blank. Your mind is a blank. Now tell me about it. Tell me what you did, how high you counted, and how long you were churning.

S: (She reported that she counted 114 strokes, and churned for ten minutes. Everything was very real to her. The churning became more difficult toward the end as the butter formed, and this slowed things down. She heard the churning, and had plenty of time. At the "stop" signal the entire scene faded from view.)

E: Show me, by counting out loud, how you counted the strokes.

S: (She counted to 60 in one minute, adding that toward the end the strokes became slowed because of the increased resistance from the butter.)

E: I'm going to wake you up by counting to ten. You will remember all about this experience and tell me about it.

S: (On waking she is again asked to give a report. Her story is similar to the above, including number of strokes counted, the time estimate and the demonstrated rate.)

In this example, then . . . the product of the demonstrated rate times the seeming duration is 600 strokes. Yet the subject insists that she took only 114 strokes, that she counted each stroke individually, and that she was occupied for the full ten minutes. When asked, posthypnotically, about the discrepancy, she had no explanation to offer [Cooper & Erickson, 1959].

Clinically, time distortion has been found to be helpful in the treatment of pain. Patients can learn to shrink an attack of pain that may have lasted for 30 minutes into sudden, intense pain 1 second in duration. Time distortion is effective in removing creative blocks, reducing stress as a result of time pressure, the treatment of dissociative disorders, and simply as an enhancement to ego functioning.

DISSOCIATION

Dissociation is a process of splitting off or isolating certain mental contents such as thoughts, memories, affects, or bodily sensations from the main body of consciousness with varying degrees of autonomy. Dissociation seems to characterize the hypnotic state more than any one phenomenon. Hilgard regards dissociation as so central to hypnosis that he named his theory of hypnosis after it. Dissociation does, in fact, seem to be part of everything that happens in hypnosis. A person recovering a traumatic event can learn to dissociate the content of the memory from the affective intensity of the memory and, if need be, recover the affect in a more gradual manner. Pain patients can learn to dissociate themselves from injured or diseased parts of the body or from the body as a whole while they exist as simply an "intellect" or "spirit" hovering over the body or in a timeless, spaceless dimension.

In hypnotherapy, dissociation is the *sin qua non* experience that facilitates the use of a parts model—that is, identifying personality parts or distinct ego states and working with them. For example, there may be a personality part that procrastinates but another part that knows how to deal with the procrastinating aspect of the self. Due to trance logic and the tolerance of incongruity of the hypnotic state, patients who tend to identify themselves too completely with their pathology can be helped to see other resources within themselves that they can experience deeply and further integrate in the trance. Hypnotherapy may be the treatment of choice for extreme forms of pathologic dissociation such as multiple personality disorder, fugue, and posttraumatic stress disorder.

AMNESIA

It is rare today for a hypnotherapy patient to develop complete amnesia for a session, though it does occur. Most patients, however, have partial spontaneous amnesias following hypnotherapy. Amnesia can be induced to varying degrees, depending on the patient and the therapeutic relationship. The use of hypnotic amnesia is indicated in situations when traumatic material needs to be contained until the patient is better able to deal with it, when conscious awareness of posthypnotic suggestions would interfere with their being carried out, or when there is any particular behavior that the patient wants to "forget about"—i.e., smoking, overeating, specific fears, nail-biting, hair-pulling, and the like.

AGE REGRESSION

Age regression is used for uncovering trauma, for the reconstruction and reintegration of personal history, and for the recalling and revivification of memories, events, and experiences. Chronically dysfunctional patients can be age-regressed back to an age before the onset of their problems, so that they can reexperience themselves when they were more healthy and functional. In selected cases, age regression is also helpful to the elderly for recapturing past events.

As with all hypnotic phenomena, age regression takes on the form of its function in the hypnotic relationship. The term *age regression* is actually a misnomer which originated from the mechanistic view of hypnosis as simply a function of suggestibility. The proof against this view is that patients rarely age-regress purely to any one chronological time. Within any regression there will be found aspects of mental functioning and behavior that are at, below, or above the "suggested" age. Regressions may remarkably focus on childhood events, but usually the patient retains an awareness of the present time. The patient is rarely amnestic to the present. Nevertheless, during genuine age regression, one often notes marked differences in a patient's behavior. The voice may change dramatically and take on the qualities and vocabulary of childhood. Likewise, drawings completed in the age-regressed state are simple and childlike as compared to the same drawings completed in the awake state or even a hypnotic state that is oriented to the adult patient's current age.

THE HYPNOTIC RELATIONSHIP

We stated earlier that hypnosis can form a link between the process orientation of analytic/psychodynamic psychotherapy and the outcome-directed mode of short-term treatment. For this reason, hypnosis is both assessment tool and change agent within a managed care context. It can readily discern which patients are candidates for short-term treatment models and which require longer-term treatment. It can unblock "stuck" treatments that might have gone unrecognized as problematic for years. How is it able to do this?

Hypnotherapy is a relational process. In fact, it requires a relationship between hypnotist and patient in order to activate or "discover" the trance.

Each trance experience is unique to the relational matrix within which it unfolds. A "good fit" between patient and therapist has enormously decisive effects on the nature of the patient's hypnotic responsiveness in terms of both the type of hypnotic phenomena experienced as well as the development of the hypnotic transference. The customary fluctuation in trance depth that occurs during and between sessions is intimately linked and governed by the corresponding changes in the relational configuration.

Our experience suggests that hypnotizability has more to do with relational factors than with strictly behavioral measures of hypnotic responsiveness. The standardized hypnotizability scales, such as the Harvard Group Scale of Hypnotic Susceptibility, Form A and the Standard Hypnotic Susceptibility Scale, Form C (the two most widely used scales) provide measures of observable behaviors only and are not relevant to clinical settings. The difference between clinical and experimental hypnosis is probably most simply contrasted by one variable—the hypnotic relationship. In a research setting, subjects are often hypnotized over a short period of time and often by different investigators. However, in a clinical setting, where the patient is hypnotized repeatedly by the same therapist over time, additional relational and psychodynamic variables develop that cannot be measured by these scales. Similarly, much of the data generated from the scales are of little value to practicing clinicians. There are patients who score very high on the scales but who, when they begin to address conflictual material, are not able to maintain a hypnotic state. On the other hand, there are those who score low on standardized tests but who use hypnosis very productively in a clinical setting.

Most often, one observes that a patient's hypnotizability will fluctuate over the course of treatment, for hypnotic responsiveness is sensitive to the shifting of transferences and the deepening of treatment issues. Just as form follows function in architecture, it is the particular function or meaning that patient and therapist have for each other that determines the form or nature of the patient's hypnotic experience. Of course, there are individual differences in hypnotic ability (Kline, 1992). The perceptual, cognitive, affective, and psychophysical changes that take place in the altered state of hypnosis vary from person to person, but the manner and extent to which a person's hypnotic potentialities can be brought forth for therapy lie in the domain of the hypnotic relationship. Many patients who are low hypnotizables benefit from hypnotherapy for this reason. It seems that in the balance of nature and nurture, where nature is an individual's capacity for hypnosis and nurture is the relationship with the therapist, it is nurture that is of prime importance. Consequently, the litmus test of a patient's likelihood of improving with hypnotherapy is whether productive treatment can be carried out during the early diagnostic uses of hypnotherapy and how this compares to the patient's productivity in the waking state. If the emphasis is on psychological productivity in hypnosis and not simply on the concept of hypnotic depth, many more patients will be found to benefit from hypnotic treatment (Kline, 1992).

In introducing hypnosis to a new patient, if the therapist is careful to initially structure the experience in ways that foster confidence and self-efficacy in the patient, a trusting therapeutic alliance will develop. This can happen very quickly in hypnosis. Whereas in conventional psychotherapy it may take months before intensified transference manifestations emerge, it can happen within a few sessions of hypnotherapy. Patients are likely to open up more quickly and easily in hypnosis—often sharing memories, fantasies, dreams, and free associations—if they are comfortable in the first few sessions. Beginning hypnotherapists may be surprised by the depth of the patient's initial material as well as its affective intensity. In hypnotic psychotherapy, there is usually less time to prepare oneself to respond to the patient's material as compared to waking-state treatment, where it emerges much more gradually. However, the hypnotherapist soon learns to see this as an advantage (Fromm & Brown, 1986). For as experience in working with altered states develops, the therapist sees that the intensity of experience, the suddenness of intimacy, and therapeutic regressions that take place in hypnosis can be remarkably well contained—that the same properties and dimensions of hypnosis that allow for rapid transference, recall, and sharing can be utilized for containment and modulation of affect, regression, dissociation, transference, and sensory experience. These procedures are less necessary with a normal or even neurotic patient population, but they may be necessary with borderline and psychotic patients. Generally if the therapist is comfortable with the depth of intimacy that results from rapid disclosure of idiosyncratic and deeply personal material, then the patient will also be comfortable. The patient deeply internalizes the therapist, incorporating him or her as a good object and associating the pleasant aspects of the altered state, such as relaxation, with the relationship to the therapist. There is an interaction between individual psychodynamic, psychoneurologic, and psychobiological functioning taking place within the patient, the result of which is an alteration in unconscious and biological information-processing patterns (Kline, 1992).

SHORT-TERM PSYCHODYNAMIC HYPNOTHERAPY

We have discussed the use of hypnosis from Freud's day and have expanded the definition of hypnotherapy based on current research and clinical work. We have described the most prominent phenomena of the hypnotic state and in doing so have also indicated that the patient maintains a locus of control. Finally, we have theorized that because hypnosis is a relational process, it can bridge those models of treatment that are process-oriented with those that are outcome-directed. For managed care, the important question is: Can hypnosis be utilized within a short-term treatment model with clearly defined outcomes? And can hypnosis do this without losing a process orientation? The answer, emphatically, is yes. The old myth that hypnotic treatment is not compatible with psychoanalytic work because it bypasses the ego is only true if one practices hypnosis to directly remove symptoms the way Freud did in the early part of his career.

Psychodynamic hypnotherapy is essentially short-term dynamic psychotherapy in which hypnosis is introduced into the treatment—usually in an auxiliary fashion—for one of the following reasons: the need to address a specific resistance; the development of a transference or alteration of an existing one; to strengthen the therapeutic alliance; to moderate affective intensity where it is overwhelming to the patient or disruptive to the therapeutic process; to support ego functions during regression; to manage disturbing or ruminating thought processes; to aid in the process of reconstruction and remembering; or to manage a symptom that may be dangerous or life-threatening to the patient (Baker, 1993).

The transference develops very rapidly in hypnosis, as do the significant conflicts that patients need to contend with to move forward with their lives. Hypnosis may evoke intense archaic primary process material, but the patient is able to experience more of it in the more relaxed and secure sense of connectedness that is present in the trance (Baker, 1993). Short-term psychodynamic hypnotherapy cannot be as comprehensive as more intensive hypnoanalytic and psychoanalytic treatments. But if patient motivation or resources preclude longer treatments, the addition of hypnosis to one's therapeutic armamentarium can be extremely valuable. Practically by definition, managed care limits resources and number of sessions for most problems for which patients seek help; therefore, short-term psychodynamic hypnotherapy is uniquely positioned to maximize the benefits within the limits imposed by managed care.

Another feature of this therapy is that hypnosis becomes less needed as the treatment proceeds. Most of the interpretation and working through is done in the waking state to maximize ego integration. During hypnosis, the patient is generally helped to gain greater access to material that is discussed in the waking state, at a later time. Ultimately the patient's ability to discuss significant areas of difficulty both in and out of trance may indicate readiness for termination (Baker, 1993).

HYPNOSIS AND MIND–BODY COMMUNICATION

Hypnosis has too often been seen as a short-term treatment for memory retrieval and abreaction. Uninformed or inexperienced clinicians who use hypnosis exclusively for memory retrieval have added to the problem. The controversy over false memory has increased anxiety about referring patients to a hypnotherapist by litigation-conscious managed care. Yet, a discussion of memory is the very place to begin considering the uses of hypnosis for somatic and psychosomatic illness.

The research on state-dependent memory as well as clinical experience has taught us that mood determines memory and not the reverse. Moods or, if you will, states of consciousness have a primacy over thoughts, cognition, fantasies, and sensory experiences. The stream of a patient's consciousness is determined by the state of her consciousness at that particular time. It follows that for change to take place in thought there must first be a more basic change in the patient's internal state.

Therapy that focuses too heavily on the verbal cognitive sphere alone often fails to recognize that cognition and intrapsychic conflicts are attached to and determined by states of consciousness—what Watkins calls ego states (Watkins & Watkins, in Keller & Heyman, 1991). Freud and Breuer wrote about this in what they called hypnoidal states (or light autohypnotic states), which some patients tend to slip into spontaneously. They believed that the patient's shift into a hypnoidal state rendered her more vulnerable to perceiving events in a traumatic way. It made good sense for them to utilize hypnosis, as they did, to reverse the effects of the traumas in their patients because they recognized the primary and overriding importance of consciousness in mental functioning. More recently, advances in biology have confirmed that memories and the affective states in which they are embedded are encoded and stored not only in the mind but in the cells of the body. The discovery of the function of information-processing substances, typically peptides, which can send traumatic messages to receptor cells in the tissues of the body, has created a whole new science of psychosomatics, which includes the study of psychoneuroimmunology and stress-related psychosomatic disorders. These advances in psychobiology are also shedding new light on the practice of psychotherapy. It seems that if state-dependent traumatic memories are being stored at the cellular level—not having reached the higher levels of verbal cortical functioning—therapy that is primarily verbal and left-hemispheric will not access the traumatic memories. Hypnosis then becomes the link between psyche and soma that allows for necessary mind-body communication to take place (Rossi & Cheek, 1988). As discussed below, this has implications in linking medical and mental health services, via hypnosis, in dealing with physical disorders, particularly those that are vulnerable to stress. Issues relevant to managed care revolve around patient selection criteria, and the idea that many patients using medical treatment they do not really need could be more effectively treated through hypnosis. Cooperative working relationships between physicians and clinical hypnotists could lead to more effective treatment plans for patients with both somatic and psychosomatic difficulties. This is the very strength that managed care purports to have—to make effective and cost-efficient treatment plans through linkage between providers. This could, in fact, be the largest area of growth for hypnotherapy utilization by managed care.

CASE DESCRIPTIONS

It is time now to turn to the practicalities of clinical work within a managed care environment. As we have pointed out, hypnosis and hypnotherapy are vastly underutilized by managed care. However, we feel that this will change once managed care is educated about hypnosis and is able to understand the true scope of this work. The following cases illustrate the varying degrees of effectiveness in work with managed care. A final case illustrates a common problem with all providers working with managed care—the abrupt and premature termination of therapy. We present it as a case that became "unstuck" through hypnotherapy and as one that perhaps would have been continued had the managed care personnel more fully understood the ongoing work of psychodynamic hypnotherapy.

A Case of Denial

Mr. C. was referred through his EAP (Employee Assistance Program) for stress reduction. However, in speaking with the EAP counselor before meeting with Mr. C., it was apparent that this was but the counselor's "hook" to get help for a client she felt was very sick indeed. The EAP had approval from the managed care insurer for 3 initial sessions and 12 sessions would be the total approved under his plan. When Mr. C. first walked into the office, he presented a shocking picture. This author has worked with many AIDS [acquired immunodeficiency syndrome] patients and he looked as if he was in a wasting stage of HIV [human immunodeficiency virus] infection. The first thing he said was "I don't have AIDS"; yet, at the very moment that our eyes met, it was clear to me that in fact he was telling me that he did. Several other comments that he made during the session as well as facts that came out during the history-taking part of the interview provided further strong evidence that Mr. C. was dealing with AIDS—that, unconsciously at least, he wanted help in finding a way to accept this diagnosis. He told me that he and his doctor "agreed" that he had Epstein–Barr syndrome. At his request, he had not been tested for HIV. The doctor was an out-of-network provider who had been Mr. C.'s doctor for several years, and Mr. C. was paying a great deal of money, it seemed, to keep the inevitable news from reaching him. He had been missing days of work and more recently began abusing alcohol. He had been referred by a manager because he had alcohol on his breath when he arrived for work on a Monday morning. He was adamant with me that I treat him for stress and said he'd been drinking because he had not been able to sleep lately. He also stated that he had no appetite and had not been eating well, and that this was the reason he'd been losing weight. I agreed to work with him initially on his sleep disorder after contracting with him not to use alcohol during our work together. I explained to him that alcohol and drug use render hypnotherapy work ineffective. Mr. C. readily agreed to this and made a second appointment that same week. It seemed to me that Mr. C. was fighting with all his might not to lose control, even as he experienced the wasting of his body, betraying his every attempt to control the progress of his illness. My intervention again shows the importance of dispelling the myth that patients have no locus of control with hypnosis.

I suggested at our next appointment that I teach him self-hypnosis so that he could obtain the sleep he so desperately needed. Mr. C. was able to experience trance quickly and easily, and I think that again this spoke to a strong motivation to keep his denial system in place. I had no intention of confronting him about his denial. The induction that I used in the office utilized time distortion. While Mr. C. was in deep trance, I suggested that each minute of real time that went by would provide as much sleep to him as one full hour. I then talked him through a full night's sleep, suggesting that he would dream and that he would remember what was only helpful and healing for him to remember of the dream. Mr. C. came out of the induction saying that he felt rested, more so than in weeks. He also stated that he'd been dreaming about food, and laughed. He'd thought of a coffee shop that he'd not been to in years. As it turned out, this was to become key information. At our third session, I again "walked" Mr. C. through a full night's sleep, and again he dreamt of food and this coffee

shop. In the meantime he had been diligently practicing self-hypnosis. In the paradoxical world of hypnosis, Mr. C. stated that he
used the self-hypnosis technique every time he thought that he
might have AIDS. In fact, I felt he was allowing himself each time
to think the unthinkable. Meanwhile, I was able to get approval
for the full 12 sessions with a diagnosis of generalized anxiety disorder. When the dream of the coffee shop came up again at the
fourth session, I wondered out loud if Mr. C. had ever thought of
going there. His appetite had improved somewhat, and I thought
perhaps, since he seemed to have such fond memories of it, he
might want to visit it. And so this is what we did in the induction: Mr. C. imagined leaving his apartment and walking through
his neighborhood, noticing many things around him, and feeling
stronger than he reported he often did these days. Yet, before
he reached the coffee shop, he turned, and it was clear that he
would go no further. Again, Mr. C. was reminded that he need
remember only what was healing for him to remember. As our
work progressed, Mr. C. did seem to find relief, stuck to his agreement not to use alcohol, and reported better sleep. He continued
to use self-hypnosis every time he thought about AIDS. He was
using self-hypnosis a great deal. We were nearing the end of the
treatment. I was becoming concerned about what would happen
to him after our work together ended. At the 11th session (the
eleventh hour?!), Mr. C. arrived and said that he didn't think that
we'd have time for hypnosis that day and that he wouldn't be
back the next week—our last session. He told me the following
story: Mr. C. had arisen last Saturday morning after a particularly restful night's sleep. He realized that he'd been dreaming
about the coffee shop again. He decided that he would go there
for breakfast. He walked through his neighborhood in much the
same way as he had during our hypnosis induction. He found the
coffee shop. He said that while he enjoyed eating there again,
he was somewhat disappointed that it didn't seem so very special. At the end of the session, he mentioned offhandedly that as
he was leaving the coffee shop, he'd noticed that the Gay Men's
Health Crisis (GMHC), an AIDS service organization, was right
down the street. And I realized that this had probably been the
very point at which he'd turned back in the hypnotic trance. He'd
been there once a couple of years ago, to accompany a friend of
his who had since died. On that day, Mr. C. had gone to the coffee
shop with his friend. This time, on the way home from the coffee shop, he walked into GMHC and picked up some literature

on their services, which included information on a group for "the worried well." He was thinking of attending. He thanked me for my help with his sleeping problem before leaving. Afterward, I thought of how unified his denial system was, and how he'd managed, I felt through the resource of his unconscious vis-à-vis our hypnosis work, to put himself in closer orbit to the services he needed—and how apt this was for him, that he would begin by going to a group for those who were worried that they might be ill. I knew that he'd found a way to get closer to what he needed to hear, and more importantly to the medical help and social support that was absolutely essential. Mr. C. had been in treatment with me for twice-a-week sessions for a month and a half. What he remembered about our treatment was that he'd been able to get some sleep and that his appetite had started to come back. It is axiomatic in hypnotherapy that the unconscious is seen as a valuable and positive resource, and that the material need not always be made conscious nor put into words.

A Case of Displacement

Ms. R., age 40, was referred by a managed care network that was knowledgeable about the use of hypnosis. Ms. R. presented as good-natured and willing to please. She said that she was having difficulty at work with a supervisor. Her blood pressure had gone up and she was recently put on medication. Her doctor, who was also knowledgeable about hypnosis, supported her idea to go to a hypnotherapist. She had heard of this author's services through a colleague and so had contacted her managed care representative for approval. She had been approved for six sessions. As Ms. R. began describing her difficulty with the supervisor, a woman older than Ms. R., her pleasant demeanor changed drastically, she became red-faced and angry, and the more she talked, the more she exhibited paranoia. She thought the supervisor was looking through her desk and tapping her phone; she even thought she saw her driving by her house one day. Of course, any of these things could be true, but Ms. R. herself, stated that when she was calmer she never thought of these things. She also said that her supervisor and she had had no problems in the past, but that in the last year or so they had had increasing difficulties. Ms. R. was particularly incensed that the supervisor actually "wagged her finger in my face" during one heated discussion. Now, every time she thought of her supervisor, all she could see was that huge finger wagging in her face. She even fantasized biting the finger off. Ms. R. was so afraid of her anger that she had been using up her sick days to stay away from the job. She now had no more left and had taken some vacation days. During the initial session and subsequently, the content of the arguments with the supervisor were explored, but nothing seemed to resonate. Ms. R. was a good hypnosis subject. However, because of the possibility that her paranoia might increase, a full hypnotic induction was not attempted until the fourth session. Again, this speaks to the need for the hypnosis subject to feel in control. It was even suggested to Ms. R. that she could focus on a particular object in the office, of her choice, and go into a trance with her eyes open. A metronome was used to assist her in doing trance with her eyes open. The regular beat appealed to her and she asked to listen to it each time she underwent an induction. Self-relaxation and guided imagery techniques were used before a full hypnotic induction was engaged. By this time, Ms. R. felt more comfortable closing her eyes. Dissociation was used in the hypnosis to help Ms. R. isolate her rage and the causes of it. She was asked to visualize her supervisor's finger wagging at her during hypnosis and, in the safety of the hypnotic trance, she was able to experience her anger. To further dissociate, she was asked to view the scene on a screen, as if she were in a movie theater. She was then told that this was one of those new "interactive movies," and she could change what was happening on the screen in any way that she'd like. In this way, Ms. R. was able both to integrate and accept the "bad" part of herself—the rageful self—as well as to practice a sense of control. In another session, Ms. R. was asked to view the "wagging finger" as very large and very close and then, on a signal from me, to shoot as far away from it as possible, as if she were a rocket, blasting off into space, and she could watch the finger growing smaller and smaller and more inconsequential. The rocket blast was a metaphor for her anger, and she was again helped to experience a sense of control. During one session, Ms. R. had a spontaneous age regression. She was a teenager and she was having an argument with her mother. Her mother started "wagging her finger at me." As soon as she said this, she began to laugh gently, while still in the trance, and while still undergoing the spontaneous age regression. This speaks again to the fact that there is still very much an observing ego in hypnotic trance, and that age regression can and does occur back and forth during the trance. In exploring her feelings about this session, Ms. R. talked about how her mother died a year ago, and it was a few months after that that she began having trouble with the supervisor. The gesture of the supervisor had only intensified her feelings and created an almost unbearable sense of grief and rage concerning her mother's death. Imagining the supervisor driving by her home brought her closer, and showed Ms. R.'s wish for her mother's presence. I was able to get an extension from her managed care plan in order to continue work on her grief and bereavement issues.

A Case of Hypnosis in Psychoanalytic Psychotherapy

A woman in her thirties entered treatment for depression and anger toward men, which threatened her work and home situations. Her background suggested that she had been severely damaged as a child by deficient parenting in a less than adequate home environment. Her father was an alcoholic who beat her and everyone else in the family and eventually left to go live with a younger woman. The patient's mother was a highly narcissistic woman who sadistically taunted and ridiculed the patient about her weight. At the time she entered treatment, Ms. K. was living with a man with whom she had a child out of wedlock. He was not willing to get married, and in addition she had just discovered that his wife had had another baby with him while he was living with the patient. This patient had many additional problems and issues to deal with.

Her lack of basic trust made it difficult for her to open up about herself. After several months of meeting on a once-per-week basis, she requested that hypnosis be used, since she was aware that this author used hypnosis. A wealth of material quickly emerged from the hypnosis sessions. She recalled many traumatic memories of abuse by her father, including a tragic scene in which he threatened her mother with a knife. Gradually, utilizing hypnosis, the patient was recapturing her past and speaking about it to another person for the first time. She was beginning to develop and express her trust and gratitude toward her male therapist for using hypnosis with her. She credited the hypnotic state with her having been able to reach more deeply into herself than she had ever done before and to face her painful past. Unfortunately, her budding sense of trust was still on tenuous ground when her benefits ran out and could not be extended. It came as a sudden shock to her when she was forced to abort her treatment. That the forced termination came at a time when she was just allowing herself to trust became an iatrogenic reenactment of her traumatic past. It had taken almost a year for her to get to this point.

In this case, the managed care insurer saw hypnosis as a therapeutic modality in itself rather than as a treatment modality informed by the psychotherapist's overall theoretical understanding. As mentioned earlier in this chapter, it is important that both hypnotherapists and managed care staff see the utilization of hypnosis in treatment as being more than the simple removal of symptoms. Hypnosis and psychodynamic hypnotherapy have the ability to quickly get at the underlying conflict that maintains the symptoms. For this reason, it is very important that the treatment not be terminated prematurely.

THE FUTURE OF HYPNOTHERAPY AND MANAGED CARE

To date, managed care has not integrated hypnosis and hypnotherapy into its treatment planning. The utilization of hypnosis is dependent upon individual case managers having their own knowledge about it. In an informal survey, the authors discovered that when asked how they felt about using hypnosis, case managers most frequently answered that it was decided on a case-by-case basis. Too many replied that it would not be approved under any circumstances. If hypnosis is to be productively utilized by managed care, there needs to be continued education. One reason why this education is lacking is that many therapists who use hypnosis in their treatment simply do not include it in their initial treatment plans. It is hidden by being described as "guided imagery," "guided relaxation," and "stress reduction." Hypnotherapists, because they use psychodynamic techniques, often avoid describing their work except as "psychotherapy." This can be problematic, to say the least, from both ethical and legal viewpoints, and it makes the hypnotherapist more vulnerable to liability claims. This is indicative of the need for more dialogue between case managers, hypnotherapists, and their professional organizations and societies.

Are there patients who are not appropriate for hypnotherapy? This question can best be answered within the context of managed care itself. As long as managed care continues to operate exclusively within a short-term model, there will be some patients who should not be treated with hypnotherapy. As in the last case outlined above, there is a danger that core issues will be uncovered that cannot be worked through because of the premature and abrupt termination of benefits. Since hypnosis often uncovers these issues and activates primitive defenses in a brief period of time, the hypnotherapist must make considered judgments about the use of hypnosis with particular patients. Patients who present with major depression, for example, would probably not be candidates for hypnotherapy unless their benefits were more open-ended. Patients who have substance abuse issues are problematic unless it is clear that they are in the early stage of disease and can effectively utilize short-term treatment and 12-step programs. (An exception would be patients who have a nicotine addiction.)

Patients who are good candidates for hypnotherapy within the managed care environment are those that have identifiable symptoms that appear at least on the surface to be self-limiting. Job stress and dissatisfaction is a common reason patients seek help, and, of course, the job dissatisfaction can often mask other issues and problems. Hypnosis can quickly identify what may be animating the job stress, and in some cases there will be a need for further treatment. The challenge for hypnotherapists as they continue to work with managed care will be to avoid the pitfall of being seen only as "symptom removers." It is important that there be a continued sense within managed care that hypnosis and hypnotherapy are important modalities that uncover core issues; that they form links between cognitive-behavioral treatment and psychoanalytic/psychodynamic treatments; and that hypnotherapy has the potential to link medical and mental health services cost-effectively and efficiently in working with psychosomatic illness.

Hypnotherapists have the ability to help patients focus their attention so that they can change their perceptions about themselves and their world. Within managed care, hypnosis needs to be given more attention, and it is important that those of us who work within this treatment model inform and educate so that managed care's perception of this profoundly useful treatment can be expanded and, ultimately, changed.

REFERENCES

Baker, E. (1993). Unpublished lecture delivered at the annual scientific meeting of the Society for Clinical and Experimental Hypnosis, Chicago.

Brown, D., & Fromm, E. (1986). *Hypnotherapy and hypnoanalysis* (pp. 3–21). Hillsdale, NJ: Erlbaum.

Cooper, L., & Erickson, M. H. (1959). *Time distortion in hypnosis* (pp. 50–51). New York: Irvington.

Freud, S. (1955). Group psychology and the analysis of the ego. In J. Strachey (Ed. and Trans.), *The standard edition of the complete psychological works of Sigmund Freud* (vol. 18, pp. 69–143). London: Hogarth Press (original work published 1921).

Fromm, E., & Nash, M. (Eds.). (1992). *Contemporary hypnosis research* (pp. 227–266). New York: Guilford Press.

Hammond, D. (Ed.). (1990) Handbook of hypnotic suggestions and metaphors (p. 2). New York and London: Norton. An American Society of Clinical Hypnosis book.

Hilgard, E. R. (1992) *Contemporary hypnosis reasearch*. E. Fromm & M. Nash (Eds). New York: Guilford.

Keller, P. A. & M. H. Heyman (Eds.), (1991). *Innovations in clinical practice: A source book*, vol. 10 (pp. 23–37). Florida: Professional Resource Exchange, Inc.

Kline, M. (1992). *Short-term dynamic hypnotherapy and hypnoanalysis* (p. 119). Springfield, IL: Charles C Thomas.

Kline, M. (1954). *Freud and hypnosis* (pp. 9–10). New York: Matrix House.

Puner, H. W. (1947). *Freud: His life and mind*. New York: Grosset and Dunlap.

Rossi, E., & Cheek, D. (1988). *Mind-body therapy: Methods of Ideodynamic healing in hypnosis*. New York: Norton.

PART III

Controversial
Issues in
Managed Care

It would be a major understatement to say that the advent of managed care has not been welcomed with enthusiasm by a large segment of the mental health profession. The most commonly expressed concern is that the cost-containment priorities integral to managed care require a short-term approach to treatment, which does not deal adequately with the severe and complex problems manifested by many patients. In addition to the charge that managed care is focused on providing treatment that is economical rather than beneficial, a number of other issues have been expressed in the current literature. These include concern about invasion of the confidentiality of the treatment relationship by the extensive reporting requirements of managed care and the ethical dilemmas raised when managed care providers have a financial investment in providing minimal services.

In this section, David Phillips examines the basic framework of professional responsibility and suggests that participation in managed care systems is beginning to significantly alter both the responsibility and areas of liability of mental health providers.

169

The group of practitioners most significantly affected by managed care is, of course, that which provides the extensive and intensive treatments of psychoanalysis and psychodynamic psychotherapy. Two experienced psychoanalysts who have been particularly critical of managed care are represented in this section. Richard Alperin discusses many of the basic incompatibilities between psychoanalytic psychotherapy and the model advocated by most managed care companies, expressing the concern that due to managed care's disregard for many important psychodynamic concepts, it is providing a form of treatment that is less effective. Joyce Edward carries forward this theme with two extended case examples that demonstrate, with particular force, the ways in which the restrictions and requirements of managed care can interfere with the process of treatment.

In the final chapter, William Herron, an author who has written extensively on the subject, offers an analysis and critique of the inadequacies of managed care on a policy level. He goes on to propose a new model for dealing more effectively with the needs of the many patients whose problems go beyond the treatment limitations of brief psychotherapy.

R.M.A.
D.G.P.

CHAPTER 9

Legal and Ethical
Issues in the Era
of Managed Care

David G. Phillips

Psychotherapists of all professional backgrounds are aware of the growing influence that managed care is having, both on their own practices and on the way that health care is delivered in the United States. Many aspects of this influence are readily apparent to practitioners in their day-to-day activity, such as that of the administrative requirements of seeing patients whose benefits are regulated by a managed care system. This chapter explores a part of the impact of managed care that is just starting to take shape and which may be less readily apparent to many psychotherapists—the impact on their legal and ethical obligations to patients. This discussion is organized in three parts: the first outlines the legal concept of the standard of care—the standard against which a practitioner is measured if he or she is accused of being negligent in the fulfillment of professional responsibilities; the second discusses one landmark case that, having completed its journey through the court system, has set a precedent in beginning to change the legal responsibility of professionals in working with managed care systems; and the third outlines some current issues regarding the ethical responsibilities of professionals in working with managed care.

THE STANDARD OF CARE

The responsibility that a professional owes to a patient is defined by a number of factors that may be more or less in agreement. Some of the key components that go into making up professional responsibility include the values and traditions of the specific profession as embodied in its code of ethics; the laws and regulations affecting the profession in the locale in which it is being practiced; and the structure and policies of the particular setting in which the professional may be working. Another factor, perhaps less familiar to many practitioners, is that of the legal concept of the "standard of care" or the "standard of the duly careful professional." This is the standard against which the actions of professionals will be evaluated in court if they are held to have been negligent in their practice—that is, if they are sued for malpractice. A number of comprehensive summaries of the elements of this standard are available (Furrow, 1980; Holder, 1983; Cohen, 1986), but since it may be unfamiliar to some readers, I will begin by reviewing its key elements.

In a general way, all adults have a legal duty to conduct themselves in a manner that is consistent with the way that any other ordinary and reasonable individual would behave in the same or similar circumstances. In a legal sense, therefore, negligent behavior consists of behavior that falls short of the standard of the "ordinary and reasonable person," which is the standard established by law for the protection of others against the unreasonable risk of harm (Cohen, 1986, pp. 251–252). In a legal action that claims negligence, the burden of proof is on the plaintiff (the individual who is claiming the negligence) and "All negligence actions are . . . predicated on the allegation that the party who claims damage was owed some duty by the other and that the duty was breached, causing injury" (Holder, 1983, p. 219).

When negligence is claimed against a professional person, the standard against which he or she is evaluated is that of the "duly careful member of the profession," a direct application of the legal concept of the "ordinary and reasonable person." A landmark court decision dating from the 1890s and quoted by Holder (1983, pp. 219–220) contains some of the central concepts that are still used in evaluating cases of professional negligence:

> . . . A physician and surgeon, by taking charge of a case, impliedly represents that he possesses, and the law places upon him the duty of possessing, that reasonable degree of learning and skill that is ordinarily possessed by physicians and surgeons in the locality in which he practices. . . . Upon consenting to treat a patient, it becomes his duty to use reasonable care and diligence in the exercise of his skill and the application of his learning to accomplish the purpose for which he was employed. He is under the further obligation to use his best judgement in exercising his skill and applying his knowledge. The law holds him liable for

an injury to his patient resulting from want of the requisite skill and knowledge or the omission to exercise reasonable care or the failure to use his best judgement. The rule in relation to learning and skill does not require the surgeon to possess that extraordinary learning and skill which belong only to a few men of rare endowments, but such as is possessed by the average member of the medical profession in good standing. . . . The rule of reasonable care and diligence does not require the use of the highest possible degree of care and to render a physician and surgeon liable, it is not enough that there has been a less degree of care than some other medical man might have bestowed, but there must be a want of ordinary and reasonable care, leading to a bad result.

As clarified in another landmark ruling in 1938, when a physician undertakes the treatment of a case he does not promise that a cure will result, and negligence cannot be assumed just because a cure does not result. By undertaking the treatment, however, there is an implied promise to use "due diligence and ordinary skill in his treatment of the patient" (Holder, 1983, pp. 219–220).

Most of the court precedents regarding professional malpractice in the United States have been in cases affecting the medical profession, dating back to the 1800s. The concepts of professional responsibility and the standard of due care would apply in a similar fashion, however, to members of other professions who might be accused of negligent practice. Psychologists and social workers, for example, would be held to the standards of practice within their respective professions.

As noted, the burden of proof is on the plaintiff to prove that he or she has been harmed by the negligent actions of the professional. In an actual case this is not a simple process, and actually four elements are required of the plaintiff in demonstrating professional malpractice.

First of all, the plaintiff must demonstrate that he or she was owed a duty of care—that, in other words, the practitioner actually undertook a professional responsibility. If the defendant did not undertake a professional responsibility in regard to the plaintiff, there can, of course, be no legal finding of negligence. If a psychotherapist is seeing a patient in ongoing therapy, it is relatively easy to determine that a professional relationship has been established and that the patient is owed a duty of care. This element is not always so easy to establish, however, as illustrated in several cases cited by Cohen (1986, pp. 253–256).

Having established the existence of a professional duty, the court would then examine the standards of the profession in order to determine how an ordinary and prudent member of that profession would have acted in the same or similar circumstances. In a malpractice case, the burden is on the plaintiff to demonstrate that the care provided by the professional fell short of that standard. Exceptions to this general rule may occur when the standard of practice is defined by law or when the court determines that the standard of the profession is too low (Cohen, 1986, p. 257). Another exception to this procedure may take place when the court invokes the doctrine of *res ipsa loquitur* ("the act speaks for itself"). Essentially this means that the practice was so clearly negligent that the court determines that expert testimony is not needed to establish that the actions of the professional fell short of the standard of the profession. An example of the kind, in which the need for expert testimony to determine the standard of the profession was obviated, is that in which a dentist had extracted the wrong tooth (Cohen, 1986, p. 257).

Establishing the standard of care in the mental health professions is not always simple, largely because there is so much genuine disagreement between practitioners of different orientations, and very little firm evidence to demonstrate which is the "correct" treatment approach. At this time, the law does not prefer any one form of treatment over another and a practitioner's professional behavior will usually be measured by the standards of his or her own treatment specialty, providing that the treatment is supported by at least a "respectable minority" of the profession (Cohen, 1986, p. 258; Holder, 1983, p. 222).

Even if the plaintiff can demonstrate that the care rendered by the professional fell short of the standard of the profession, he or she can recover damages only by also establishing "proximate cause." This means that the plaintiff must prove that he or she was injured *and* that the negligent practice of the professional was the cause of that injury: "He cannot recover damages unless he can also prove that the negligence caused him injuries which would not have occurred in its absence" (Holder, 1983, p. 228). The establishment of proximate cause, which really requires two points, comprises the third and fourth elements that must be demonstrated by the plaintiff in proving a case of professional negligence. Even if the professional was flagrantly negligent, there can be no recovery of damages unless this practice can be shown to have caused injuries to the plaintiff. This concept is illustrated in a somewhat startling case cited by Holder (1983, p. 229): "An automobile accident victim had a broken leg. By mistake, the cast was put on the wrong leg and the error was not discovered for 10 days. Since the residual stiffness of the leg was as likely to have been caused by the accident itself as it was by the error, no proximate cause of damage was shown against the orthopedist."

A hypothetical example may clarify how the concept of the standard of due care may work in actual practice and how a professional may be judged in a specific case. A professional is not necessarily guilty of negligence simply because a patient does not improve as a result of the treatment. In undertaking the treatment, the professional does not promise to bring about a cure but is simply required to use due diligence and ordinary skill with the patient. An unsuccessful outcome is never, in and of itself, proof of negligence. But while the standard of due care does not suggest that the professional has been negligent when the patient does not improve, the concepts of "due diligence and ordinary skill" may make other demands on the practitioner. If a case is not going well, the standard of due care may require the professional to consult with other practitioners; to refer the patient for further evaluation and possible treatment to a specialist who may be able to help; and/or to consult with another practitioner if he or she knows or should know that the methods of dealing with the case are proving to be ineffectual (Holder, 1983, p. 223).

In the next part we will examine, in some detail, a landmark managed care case that has begun to establish a legal precedent, defining new obligations for practitioners working in those systems.

THE WICKLINE CASE AND THE
DUTY OF ECONOMIC ADVOCACY

A number of cases in various stages of the legal process have challenged aspects of the policies and practices of managed care and utilization review companies (Tischler, 1990; Sederer, 1992; Appelbaum, 1993). The most significant case, however, which has already begun to alter *legal* precedents for practitioners working with managed care companies, is that of *Wickline v. State of California*. Although this case does not involve psychiatric illness, it is considered a landmark in beginning to establish new obligations for both practitioners and utilization review organizations (Sederer, 1992, p. 1157).

Lois Wickline was covered by Medi-Cal (Medicaid of California) and in 1976 received utilization review approval for admission to a hospital for surgical treatment of an obstruction of the terminal aorta, a vessel in the abdomen, which is a major source of blood to the lower extremities. In this procedure the section of the obstructed blood vessel is replaced, but on the day of her surgery Mrs. Wickline needed a second operation for a blood clot that had formed in the graft. Five days later she required another procedure (lumbar sympathectomy) for pain secondary to vessel spasm. Her insurance approval was due to expire 4 days later, and her doctor asked for an 8-day extension of her hospitalization. The utilization review organization approved a 4-day extension, which her doctors did not appeal, and she was discharged after the 4-day extension. Nine days later she required emergency readmission for clotting and infection at the site of the graft. Subsequent complications required Mrs. Wickline to endure first below-the-knee and then above-the-knee amputations of her right leg.

Mrs. Wickline did not seek damages from her doctors but did sue the State of California and its medical review organization, alleging that she had been injured by the decision of the Medi-Cal consultant, which had denied coverage for necessary postoperative care in the hospital and had led to her premature discharge. In the first level of the legal process, in trial court, she was awarded $500,000. The verdict was appealed, and the appellate court both dismissed the State as a defendant and reversed the verdict of the lower court. The Supreme Court of California then declined to hear the case, which rendered the decision of the appellate court final.

The reader may well be shocked to see that an individual who had suffered so much did not receive at least some financial compensation. The reason was that since Mrs. Wickline's doctors *had not appealed* the utilization review decision, the court ruled that Medi-Cal had never had a chance to review their concerns about her discharge. Even though Mrs. Wickline failed to win anything from her case, two "critical" lessons for practitioners emerge from this case (Sederer, 1992, p. 1158).

The first conclusion is the legal precedent that a tort (a wrongful act or injury for which a civil suit can be brought) can derive from medically inappropriate decisions stemming from cost-containment practices. In the language of the Court of Appeals:

> The patient who requires treatment and who is harmed when care which should have been provided is not provided should recover for the injuries suffered from all those responsible for the deprivation of such care, including, when appropriate, health care payers. Third party payers of health care services can be held legally accountable when medically inappropriate decisions result from defects in the design or implementation of cost containment mechanisms as, for example when appeals made on a patient's behalf for medical or hospital care are arbitrarily ignored or unreasonably disregarded or overridden [cited in Tischler, 1990, p. 971].

So the first lesson of the Wickline case is that managed care and utilization review companies can potentially be held liable when patients are harmed because of premature termination of benefits. What, however, does all this mean for practitioners working with managed care?

This is the second lesson of this case, which can also be stated in the language of the court: "The physician who complies without protest with the limitations imposed by a third party payor when his medical judgement dictates otherwise, cannot avoid his ultimate responsibility for the patient's care" (cited in Appelbaum, 1993, p. 253). No liability was imposed on Mrs. Wickline's doctors, who were not sued, but the language of the court strongly suggests that such a penalty could have been imposed. The managed care or utilization review company *can* be held liable if a patient is harmed because of premature termination of benefits, but only if they have been made fully aware of the seriousness of the situation by the provider. The provider who fails to fulfill this part of the responsibility to the patient may well be the one held to be liable for harm that is done.

Commentators on the Wickline case have suggested that it states a new "practice guideline" for physicians (and, by implication, other health care professionals working with managed care organizations)—a duty of "economic advocacy," the responsibility to appeal adverse decisions by the managed care company that may harm the patient (Morreim, 1991; Sederer, 1992; Appelbaum, 1993). Morreim has been particularly forceful in her proposal that the physician act as an economic advocate, helping the patient to obtain all the resources to which he or she is legally and economically entitled. She has stated, for example, that "Such advocacy is pertinent under the principle of self-determination, because in many instances a person initiates a physician–patient relationship as a means by which to reach a goal or implement a plan that he or she cannot attain alone. . . . In some instances, the patient also needs the physician's vigorous lobbying efforts, such as to persuade recalcitrant utilization reviewers of the necessity of treatment" (Morreim, 1991, p. 292).

But even if we accept such a duty of "economic advocacy," a number of further questions remain, as also suggested in the writings of Appelbaum (1993) and Wolf (1994). Must, for instance, every case be appealed, and how far should such appeals be carried? Managed care companies typically have several levels in the appeals process, and going through this process is often cumbersome and time-consuming for practitioners who are already overwhelmed with administrative obligations. Furthermore, providers who continually appeal adverse decisions are not free of personal risk. They may well be identified as "unfriendly" to managed care, with subsequent negative consequences to their professional and economic well-being. In addition, some managed care contracts require providers to share in the costs of appeals that may be taken to an independent third party such as the American Arbitration Association.

Another question that has been raised is whether the likelihood of success should affect the duty to appeal (Appelbaum, 1993, p. 253). In Virginia, for example, Blue Cross/Blue Shield has a 4.6% rate of approving appeals. If the practitioner believes that there is such a slight chance of success, is there a duty to appeal every adverse decision?

On the other hand, managed care entities are beginning to try to avoid liability by never discontinuing coverage when a caregiver feels strongly that further treatment is needed. Their lawyers are advising them to approve continued care for at least an interim period; therefore at least in the short run, appeals by practitioners are likely to be more meaningful (Appelbaum, 1993, p. 253).

Wolf (1994) has criticized existing codes of medical ethics for not providing adequate guidance for physicians who might want to undertake a responsibility of economic advocacy for their patients; she has offered a conceptual framework for guiding them in this type of activity. A similar criticism could have been made of other ethical codes that make general statements about a duty of advocacy for clients without providing a specific plan of action. It may well be, however, that professional codes are not the proper place to specify such detailed plans of action and that they will inevitably be developed in other writings.

Appelbaum, for example, has offered a number of pragmatic suggestions on this subject "from a clinician's point of view" (1993, p. 253):

> At least an initial appeal of adverse decisions should be undertaken when a clinician believes that the treatment in question is necessary for a patient's well-being. Further levels of appeal probably should be pursued only after consultation with the patient, taking into consideration the likelihood of success, whether the patient still desires to proceed with treatment, and the availability of alternative means of paying for care.

ADDITIONAL ETHICAL ISSUES
IN WORK WITH MANAGED CARE

As previously noted, authors on ethics are beginning to review codes of ethics and to call on professions to revise those codes to deal with the new dilemmas and obligations that occur in work with managed care systems (Morreim, 1991; Wolf, 1994). This emerging literature is beginning to refer to two possible ethical duties for professionals working within those systems, although the existence of these duties has not yet been ruled on by any court (Appelbaum, 1993, p. 254).

Informed Consent and the Right of Economic Disclosure

The doctrine of informed consent to treatment has been developing since at least the late eighteenth century in the English case of *Slater v. Baker and Stapleton* (cited in Malcolm, 1988, chap. 6). The plaintiff in this case had hired the defendants to remove the bandages from his leg, which had previously been broken and set. In addition, however, the defendants attempted to straighten the plaintiff's "crooked" leg and he sued, claiming that he had been injured as a result of their negligence. One of the defendants was considered an "eminent" and "celebrated" surgeon, but both he and his assistant were found liable for having detached a callus that had formed over the plaintiff's partially healed facture without first obtaining his consent. The jury found the defendants negligent and awarded the plaintiff the very large sum of 500 pounds.

The court in the *Slater* case affirmed the judgment, pointing out that the practice of obtaining a patient's consent before proceeding with treatment was customary among surgeons in England—partially basing the duty, therefore, on the concept of the prevailing standard of care. In addition, the *Slater* court pointed out a further justification for imposing this duty on the surgeon, stating "it is reasonable that a patient should be told what is about to be done to him, that he may take courage and put himself in such a situation as to enable him to undergo the operation" (Malcolm, 1988, p. 62).

When informed consent cases began to appear in the beginning of this century, they were based on a different rationale:

> The doctrine of informed consent, as it appeared in those cases, was rooted in the common law tort of battery. In general, the tort of battery is concerned with two interests: physical (i.e., that the body be free from harmful contacts) and dignitary (i.e., that the body be free from unwanted or offensive contacts) [Malcolm, 1988, p. 62].

Probably the most famous statement of the doctrine of informed consent was the summation of Justice Benjamin Cardozo: "Every human being of adult years and sound mind has a right to determine what shall be done with his own body" (Malcolm, 1988, p. 62).

In early cases, the patient's simple consent to treatment was seen as adequate, but gradually a concept that requires an "informed consent" has developed. Courts have affirmed with increasing force the right of patients to receive the information necessary to make their own medical decisions.

This affirmation of the patient's right to self-determination has been based not on what other physicians disclose (an important exception to the concept of the standard of care) but on the right of the patient to know the material facts that will be needed to make appropriate treatment decisions (Morreim, 1991, p. 290).

The importance of this right, for both patients and research subjects, received further impetus from the Nuremberg war crimes trials in which it was revealed that prisoners in concentration camps had been subjected to horrible tortures in the name of "scientific research," and currently the "issue of informed consent has probably received more attention than any other issue in biomedical ethics" (Beauchamp & Childress, 1989, p. 74). In current writings the focus on informed consent has shifted from a discussion of the physician's duty to disclose, to a focus on the elements required for the patient to understand and to give a meaningful consent (Beauchamp & Childress, 1989, p. 74).

A number of valuable discussions on informed consent are available (Beauchamp & Childress, 1989, chap. 3; Furrow, 1980, chap. 9; Morreim, 1991), but this topic has received relatively little attention in the psychotherapy literature. There is, however, general agreement on the elements required in any genuine informed consent process: (1) the person giving the consent must be competent to give a meaningful consent; (2) the relevant information must be disclosed in such a way that the person giving the consent can understand it; (3) the person giving the consent must understand the risks and benefits of the treatment being proposed, the risks and benefits of alternative treatments, and the risks and benefits of no treatment; and (4) the consent that is given must be truly voluntary (Beauchamp & Childress, 1989, chap. 3).

The codes of ethics of the major professions and professional organizations reflect the duty to obtain an informed consent to treatment—as stated, for instance in the Code of the National Federation of Societies for Clinical Social Work: "Clinical social workers inform clients of the extent and nature of services available to them as well as the limits, rights, opportunities, and obligations associated with service which might affect the client's decision to enter into or continue the relationship" (1988, p. 11).

Authors such as Morreim (1991) and Wolf (1994) have argued, however, that the new economic realities of managed care require the professions to revise both their codes and their concepts of informed consent. Morreim, in particular, raises a number of troubling questions in stating that profound changes in medical economics give rise to a new duty of economic disclosure, which "requires physicians to discuss such matters as prices, conflicts of interest, and economically prompted deviations below the standard of care" (Morreim, 1991, p. 280). The point about "conflicts of interest" seems to indicate Morreim's belief that, for instance, practitioners working in certain types of HMO arrangements need to inform their patients of the professional's possible financial benefit in providing minimal treatment. In the final point, Morreim is saying that practitioners in managed care arrangements often know that economic constraints will prevent them from providing the treatment that they feel the patient really needs, and the patient needs to know this too.

Space does not permit a fuller discussion of some of these complex and troubling issues, but Appelbaum (1993, p. 254) does offer a clear and specific outline of what a duty of economic disclosure under managed care might include:

> At the initiation of therapy, clinicians might want to discuss with patients the potential effects of managed care on the course of treatment, including the possibility that payment for therapy might be terminated before either the patient or the clinician believes that the goals of treatment have been achieved. Patients who are about to embark on therapy involving painful self-disclosure and the activation of disturbing affects might well find such information important to their decision to proceed. Disclosure of the nature and extent of information that may have to be released to managed care reviewers may also be useful to patients. When further coverage is denied, clinicians will probably need to enter into a full discussion of patient's options.

The Duty to Continue Treatment

Managed care has developed a number of strategies to meet cost-containment goals by placing external limits on the length of therapy. These mechanisms include placing controls on the number of sessions that will be allowed, placing dollar caps on the mental health benefits that will be allowed, and the process of utilization review in which the progress of the treatment toward meeting its goals is regularly evaluated (Stern, 1993, p. 162).

Stern goes on to point out that there is no question that short-term therapy is the treatment of choice for many patients and that many other patients "self-select" short-term treatment through early termination. The key question, however, is whether short-term therapy is the treatment of choice for *everyone*. He notes (1993, p. 168) that brief therapy was never intended as a universal mode of treatment, and its early developers were very conservative in selecting appropriate candidates for it. In addition, the research on psychotherapy outcomes suggests that patients who remain in treatment for a longer duration do so because they do not feel sufficiently improved to stop (Stern, 1993, p. 171).

While the mandating of brief therapy is appropriate for many patients and therapists, it raises a complex legal and ethical problem for many others. The issue, quite simply, is that many therapists will be in the position of having to offer a treatment that they believe not to be the most effective or in the best interests of the patient. We have seen in our earlier discussion that these limitations of treatment require an increased duty of disclosure by professionals, but the questions go far beyond those of informed consent to treatment. Lynch (1994, p. 151) wrote in the context of rehabilitation medicine, but he asked questions that any other practitioner might raise: "As professionals we see the patient in need of a certain course of therapy. How do we fulfill our professional duties and obligations to the patient and at the same time comply with insurance regulations?" The answers to these questions are still quite unclear, from both a legal and an ethical perspective.

In writing on this topic, Appelbaum (1993, p. 254) points out that authorities would agree that there is a duty to continue treatment when the professional believes that an emergency situation exists. At the same time, this is an unlikely scenario, since most insurance coverage would continue in the case of an emergency.

The nature of the therapist's obligation to continue treatment in nonemergency situations is less clear, although Appelbaum points out that there are court decisions indicating that clinicians and hospitals must provide all necessary care once they accept a patient for treatment. In one recent case, a group of psychiatrists attempted to terminate a managed care agreement alleging that it had negative effects on patient care. In rejecting their claim, the court stated: "Whether or not the proposed treatment is approved, the physician retains the right and indeed the ethical and legal obligation to provide appropriate treatment to the patient" (*Varol v. Blue Cross and Blue Shield of Michigan*, 1989; cited in Appelbaum, 1993, p. 254).

Professional codes of ethics deal with the question of termination of therapy and usually focus on the welfare of the patient as being the primary consideration in making this decision. A typical example is found in the Code of the National Association of Social Workers: "The social worker should terminate service to clients, and professional relationships with them, when such service and relationships are no longer required or no longer serve the clients' needs or interests" (1993, p. 5). Professional codes and the standard of care always require an appropriate and responsible termination process, and such a process would include a review of alternative means of obtaining needed treatment.

The fact is that practitioners have rarely been able to provide optimal care for their patients, and the provision of continued treatment when insurance benefits have expired has long been a problem. The legal concept of the standard of care does not refer to a rigid set of rules but rather to a broad guideline for good practice. With some exceptions, such as the doctrine of informed consent, good practice means what is usual and customary within the field. It may well be that one of the most significant long-term effects of managed care, and the general trend toward increasing cost containment, will be to reduce the standard of care for practice in many professional fields (Hirshfeld, 1990). Evidently, this has already started to happen in the field of rehabilitation medicine:

> Managed care has had a significant impact on how providers rehabilitate patients. Experts say the goal of treatment used to be restoring complete physical and cognitive function in a patient. Now it is simply improving the patient's physical functioning and doing the best in a limited amount of time to correct the cognitive effects of a stroke or injury. Reimbursement for stroke patients and patients with spinal cord injuries and traumatic brain injury has dropped from an average of 12 weeks in the 1980s to six to eight weeks in the 1990s [Lynch, 1994, p. 151].

As Applebaum has pointed out (1993, p. 254), it is unrealistic to expect clinicians and hospitals to provide unlimited amounts of uncompensated care, and it is not likely that such a responsibility will be expected as a result of new cost-containment measures. Professionals may engage in economic advocacy for individual patients as well as to change policies of managed care organizations. The welfare of the individual patient is still the primary responsibility of the professional, but this duty can be discharged in a number of ways, as illustrated by the recent guidelines on working with managed care of the National Association of Social Workers (1993, p. 10):

> When managed care organizations determine that they will no longer authorize payment for services by virtue of benefit limits, the social worker has the obligation to assure that appropriate services are made available to the client. The options include acceptance of private payment at a regular or reduced fee, pro bono services, referral to alternative treatment sources, or termination of treatment.

REFERENCES

American Board of Examiners in Clinical Social Work (1993). *Guidelines for establishing standards for care in clinical social work practice.*

Appelbaum, P. (1993). Legal liability and managed care. *American Psychologist, 48,* 251–257.

Bennet, M. (1988). The greening of the HMO: Implications for prepaid psychiatry. *American Journal of Psychiatry, 145,* 1544–1549.

Beauchamp, T. & Childress, J. (1989). *Principles of bio-medical Ethics* (3rd ed.). New York: Oxford University Press.

Cohen, R. J. (1986). The professional liability of behavioral scientists: An overview. In L. Everstine & D. Everstine (Eds.). *Psychotherapy and the law.* New York: Grune & Stratton.

Furrow, B. (1980). *Malpractice in psychotherapy.* Lexington Books.

Gabbard, G., Tetjuro, T., Davidson, J. et al. (1991). A psychodynamic perspective on the clinical impact of insurance review. *American Journal of Psychiatry, 148,* 318–323.

Hirshfeld, E. (1990). Economic considerations in treatment decisions and the standard of care in medical malpractice litigation. *Journal of the American Medical Association, 264,* 2004–2012.

Holder, A. (1983). The duty of care. In N. Abrams & M. Buckner (Eds.) *Medical ethics.* Cambridge, MA: MIT Press.

Lynch, J. (1994). (Cited in) Managed care poses ethical dilemmas in rehab medicine; *Medical Ethics Advisor. 10,* 1151–1153.

Malcolm, J. (1988). *Treatment choices and informed consent.* Springfield, IL: Charles C Thomas.

Morreim, E. H. (1991). Economic disclosure and economic advocacy: New duties in the medical standard of care. *Journal of Legal Medicine, 12,* 275–329.

National Association of Social Workers (1993). *Code of Ethics.*

National Association of Social Workers (1993). The social work perspective on managed care for mental health and substance abuse treatment.

National Federation of Societies for Clinical Social Work (1988). *Code of Ethics.*

Norquist, G., & Wells, K. (1991). How do HMOs reduce outpatient mental health care costs? *American Journal of Psychiatry, 148,* 96–101.

Sederer, L. (1992). Judicial and legislative responses to cost containment; *American Journal of Psychiatry, 149,* 1157–1161.

Sharfstein, S., Stoline, A., & Goldman, H. (1993). Psychiatric care and health insurance reform. *American Journal of Psychiatry, 150,* 7–18.

Stern, S. (1993). Managed care, brief therapy, and therapeutic integrity. *Psychotherapy, 30,* 162–175.

Tischler, G. (1990). Utilization management of mental health services by private third parties. *American Journal of Psychiatry, 147,* 967–973.

Wolf, S. (1994). Health care reform and the future of physician ethics. *Hastings Center Report, 24,* 28–41.

CHAPTER 10

Is Psychoanalytically Oriented Psychotherapy Compatible with Managed Care?

Richard M. Alperin

Over the past decade we have witnessed the growth of managed care, which has drastically altered the delivery, definition, and outcome of the psychotherapy that many patients receive (Bozzuto, 1992). While some mental health professionals have welcomed this trend with hopes that referrals from managed care companies will enhance their private practices, many have not responded favorably. This is particularly true of psychodynamically oriented practitioners whose approach to treatment often seems antithetical to that espoused by most managed care companies. These practitioners feel that the greater majority of managed care companies are biased against psychodynamic psychotherapy, so that their practice is often incompatible with managed care. To determine whether these concerns are justified, some of the basic tenets of psychoanalytic° psychotherapy will be reviewed and then compared to those of managed care in an attempt to answer the question, "Is psychoanalytically oriented psychotherapy compatible with managed care?"

°The terms *psychoanalytic* and *psychodynamic* are used interchangeably in this chapter.

THE THERAPEUTIC RELATIONSHIP

It is generally believed by most psychoanalytic practitioners that the majority of patients today—unlike Freud's psychoneurotic patients, who presumably had reached high levels of ego integration—are suffering from problems that originated during the preoedipal period (Blanck & Blanck, 1974; Giovacchinni, 1979; Kernberg, 1975; Kohut, 1984; Masterson, 1976). With these patients especially, the curative value of the therapeutic relationship cannot be overemphasized. A framework considered useful for understanding this relationship is that of the "holding environment," similar to the holding of the infant by the good parent (Winnicott, 1965). Essential for gorwth is that the patient gradually perceive this environment as safe, secure, and trustworthy.

To help these patients feel protected within this environment, a "frame" containing the ground rules for the analysis is mandatory (Bleger, 1967; Langs, 1982). Critical to its formation is an explicit initial contract between therapist and patient about the frequency of sessions, regular appointment time(s), money arrangements, and whether the therapy is a brief model or open-ended.

Since so many of our patients are suffering from histories of inconsistent and unreliable parenting, having even felt that their presence within their home was conditional, a secure and steady frame is critical. Having never achieved object constancy, most of these patients have intense fears of separation and loss; their greatest transferential fear is that their therapists will also abandon them. To relieve them of these fears, verbal interventions are far less effective than the establishment of a benign holding environment characterized by consistency, predictability, and reliability. The patient should also experience the holding environment as a setting where nothing is demanded of him or her, so as to ensure continued care and acceptance (Cohen & Sherwood, 1991).

Establishing such an environment with most patients usually takes well over a year (Modell, 1976); this is often an impossibility under managed care, since managed care plans usually allow for no more than 20 sessions of psychotherapy. However, even when the managed care company does not explicitly limit the number of sessions, achieving such an environment still remains unfeasible, since the therapist cannot set up a secure frame with the patient that ensures the continuity of treatment. Because of frequent case reviews (usually every 5 to 10 sessions) to determine the necessity for further treatment, there is constantly the threat that the therapy will be terminated abruptly. As a result, patients experience uncertainty and anxiety similar to that which they experienced in the past. This limits their emotional involvement in the therapeutic process, frequently preventing them from sharing anything but superficial concerns. Consequently, the effectiveness of the therapy is seriously undermined.

Another aspect of the therapeutic frame that is of great importance to the analytic therapist is the arrangement of fees. While most no longer subscribe to Freud's original notion that the patient's financial sacrifice is a necessary incentive for successful treatment (Meehan, 1994), almost all attach great emotional and symbolic meaning to the exchange of money. Therefore it is strongly recommended that even when the patient receives insurance reimbursements, the money be sent directly to the patient, with the patient taking full responsibility for the direct payment of fees to the therapist (Goldesohn, 1986). Because of the policy of most managed care companies that the insurance company pays the provider directly for his or her services and that the patient is responsible for a much smaller co-payment, a beneficial aspect of the therapeutic process is interfered with, as the therapeutic dyad is deprived of an excellent opportunity to examine certain conflicts within the relationship (DiBella, 1986).

Also considered essential by psychodynamic practitioners for the establishment of a safe and secure therapeutic environment is complete privacy and confidentiality. As Langs (1982) states:

> Essential here is the therapist's offer of a psychotherapeutic space that is exclusively the patient's and into which no one else is permitted, directly or indirectly, to the greatest extent possible. This implies that actual intrusions of third parties, the offer of information to outsiders, are all to be excluded. In this way, the therapist indicates to the patient that he or she is prepared to offer the safety of a totally private and confidential relationship and that he or she is capable as well of being the sole individual who will attempt to cure the patient of emotional ills [p. 475].

Those psychotherapists offering services under managed care cannot provide their patients with the privacy and confidentiality considered necessary for psychotherapeutic success, since managed care companies require the therapist to reveal detailed information about their patients and the treatment for continued coverage. It should be noted that Langs (1982) believes that the sharing of any information whatsoever with an insurance company, even when the patient expresses a manifest desire for the therapist to do so, is injurious to the treatment, because on an unconscious level, it generates an image of the therapist as untrustworthy and the therapeutic environment as threatening and unsafe.

Particularly with those mistrustful patients with paranoid features or those reluctant to seek help in the first place, sharing this information may be destructive to the therapeutic alliance. Kernberg and his colleagues (1989) feel that this disclosure to an insurance company may prove disruptive to the treatment and require many sessions to work through. This is a luxury, however, which very few patients and therapists can afford under managed care, since its therapy is usually short-term.

PSYCHOPATHOLOGY AND ITS TREATMENT

During its early development, psychoanalysis was primarily concerned with the formation and cure of neurotic symptomatology. It was Freud's discovery of the concept of resistance that moved psychoanalysis beyond symptoms to the treatment of character. The publication of Wilhelm Reich's book *Character Analysis* (1933) heralded a transition from an analysis of symptoms to an analysis of character that continues to be of central concern to psychodynamically oriented practitioners. General psychiatry, in concordance with psychodynamic therapy, also considers the diagnosis and treatment of character pathology significant, as evidenced by the inclusion of an Axis II diagnosis and 10 major character disorders in the fourth edition of the *Diagnostic and Statistical Manual of Mental Disorders* (A.P.A., 1994).

Contrary to this long-established concern with character pathology and its treatment, managed care tends to ignore character by virtue of its focus only on the eradication of symptoms. Because of their strong bias against clinical issues related to character, expert managed care providers recommend against even offering managed care an Axis II diagnosis (Goodman et al., 1992).

There is also a wide disparity between psychodynamic psychotherapy and managed care in the understanding of symptomatology and the treatment of these problems. Managed care seems to be exclusively concerned only with those symptoms resulting in an *identifiable* impairment in functioning. Disregarded are intrapsychic symptoms that are not always observable in daily functioning, such as a poor self-esteem or sadness. Also disregarded are the underlying intrapsychic conflicts creating these symptoms. This totally goes against Freud's belief that assessing behavior and symptomatology purely on the basis of overt conduct and conscious motive constituted a superficial understanding of human behavior, and that not until the unconscious motive for behavior was discovered could a person be properly understood (Josephs, 1992).

Because only symptoms and their behavioral manifestations are of concern to most managed care companies, the majority recommend only brief, crisis-oriented therapy of 20 sessions or less. This has recently led to a proliferation of literature in the field of mental health recommending a variety of short-term treatment approaches; there is even a text that asserts that a patient can be adequately helped within a single session (Talman, 1990).

Managed care justifies its bias toward short-term therapy with usage data research demonstrating that most patients discontinue treatment well before 20 sessions, with the median number being 5 to 6 sessions (Garfield, 1978). However, the studies cited in this research are not necessarily applicable to the practice of psychoanalytically oriented psychotherapy, since they provide no data whatsoever on the orientation or qualifications of the therapists in the sample and whether they received a personal analysis, psychoanalytically oriented supervision, and relevant postgraduate coursework—training considered indispensable for the competent practice of psychoanalytically oriented psychotherapy (Alperin & Hollman, 1992).

Based upon their own experience and practice, many psychodynamically oriented practitioners dispute this finding. As a matter of fact, when the above statistic was quoted at a meeting I attended sponsored by a managed care company, all of the practitioners present stated that this attendance figure was contrary to their clinical experience; they strongly agreed that more than 20 sessions were necessary to alleviate most patients' symptoms. Even a psychologist representing many of his colleagues practicing behavior therapy, stated that while he was very effective and adept in the practice of short-term therapy, he too doubted that symptoms could be alleviated with the majority of patients in so few sessions. Furthermore, statistics on how quickly patients discontinue treatment should not be taken as prescriptions for how long treatment should last, since a significant number of patients discontinue treatment without being adequately helped.

Managed care companies also support their preference for short-term therapy with their assertion that long-term therapy is no more effective than short-term therapy. While, historically, psychoanalytic practitioners have eschewed empirical research in favor of findings from the study of individual cases, there are numerous outcome studies that document the efficacy of long-term psychoanalytic treatment (Applebaum, 1977; Bachrach et al., 1985; Kernberg et al., 1972; Wallerstein, 1986; Weber et al., 1985). There are, unfortunately, no studies that clearly show a difference between short- and long-term therapy (Budman & Gurman, 1988). The paucity of research examining this issue is, as Weinberg (1994) correctly concludes, no one's fault but our own.

While many psychodynamic practitioners believe that short-term psychotherapy is effective for certain patients, very few believe it is appropriate for the entire clinical population, as some managed care companies suggest. After all, its innovators (i.e., Davenloo, 1978; Mann, 1973; Marmor, 1979; Sifneos, 1978) were extremely conservative as to who is an appropriate candidate for such treatment and never intended it to be a universal mode of treatment. The application of this model for *all* clinical cases, especially those with severe preoedipal pathology, is inappropriate and might even be destructive. That is why Stern (1993) suggests that undertaking this form of treatment without criteria for selection is a violation of the therapist's integrity.

For those patients who fail to quickly respond to this short-term model, many managed care companies feel that medication is warranted rather than longer-term therapy. While there are instances when most psychoanalytic psychotherapists feel that medication is warranted, as when the patient cannot function or is unable to derive benefit from therapy, it is rarely viewed as a real solution. Rather, the psychodynamic practitioner cautiously deliberates upon its meaning as well as its effect on the treatment, since it might interfere with the patient's transference and reduce the chances of clinical success (Horner, 1991; Spotnitz, 1985).

Many managed care companies are also biased toward behavior therapy, as evidenced by their emphasis on a behavioral language to describe impairments in functioning, the application of specific behavioral interventions, and operationally recorded outcome measures. Traditional psychoanalytic concerns with transference and resistance are disregarded in the "common behavioral language of treatment" of managed care (Goodman et al., 1992, p. 22), and specific behavioral interventions such as stress management and assertiveness training are preferred over those psychoanalytic techniques designed to make the unconscious conscious.

In response to this bias, some psychodynamic practitioners recommend to their colleagues that, for the purposes of managed care, they simply translate what they do into behavioral terminology. While for some this advice may be easy to implement, the vast majority feel it is a distortion of the therapeutic process and demeaning to the practice of psychodynamic psychotherapy.

THE IMPACT OF UTILIZATION REVIEW ON THE THERAPEUTIC PROCESS

Psychodynamic practitioners are well aware that an outside observer can have a profound impact on the two-person system of patient and therapist. This is carefully documented in the literature on the parallel process in supervision (Caligor, 1981; Fiscalini, 1985). Since it concludes that the nature and quality of the supervisory relationship affects and influences the therapeutic relationship, psychoanalytic supervision should always be conducted with considerable tact and sensitivity to the supervisee's feelings.

Like supervisors, managed care's case reviewers are an omnipotent force in the treatment process. Often they make the referral, require a treatment plan in the diagnostic phase, and closely monitor the patient's progress. Besides determining the extent of the patient's psychotherapy benefits and the therapist's compensation for the treatment, they also evaluate the therapist's performance, which determines the company's future referrals to that therapist. Because managed care's review process has such a profound impact upon the treatment, like supervision, it follows the Heisenberg principle, which states that the act of observing and measuring has an unaccountable effect on the field at the moment of scrutiny (Marshall & Marshall, 1988).

Although case reviewers are supposed to be concerned about patient care as well as containment of costs, most often they behave only with the latter goal in mind. As a result, therapists often find them critical and unempathic—even a major source of difficulty in their work with patients (Bozzuto, 1992; Edward, 1992).

Many therapists report that case reviewers are frequently impatient with them when their patients fail to improve immediately and assume an attitude of superiority, as if they had greater expertise and could function more effectively with that patient. Other outside observers, such as supervisors or participants in a case seminar, are also susceptible to this trap: since they have no personal contact with the patient, they are not confronted with the patient's idiosyncrasies and not subjected to the same countertransferential pulls as is the therapist. At this different level of abstraction, it is easy for the reviewer to develop unrealistic expectations and illusions of omniscience.

Unlike those who conduct psychoanalytic supervision properly, some managed care case reviewers seem to be impervious to the fact that their behavior may prove upsetting to the therapist and may in various ways—particularly through the parallel process—prove destructive to the therapy itself. Thus the reviewer has the potential of becoming a major source of difficulty in the relationship between therapist and patient. One common way in which I have seen this reenacted among supervisees is for the therapist to become impatient, demanding that the patient improve at an impossible rate, forgetting that the patient is developmentally arrested and not always capable of mature functioning. Since this can be a repetition of the patient's past—when he or she was regarded as bad and inadequate rather than a person with legitimate problems—when therapists are cast in this role, patients feel misunderstood and narcissistically wounded (Gabbard et al., 1991) and the progress of treatment is stunted.

Psychoanalytic supervisors are very cognizant of the fact that their supervisees are only human and, like everyone else, will resort to certain defense mechanisms when feeling pressured and anxious. The supervisory process itself is anxiety-producing, as is the therapist's daily work, since he or she is the target for much of the patients' anger and hostility. Rather than complicate this anxiety, good supervision aims at reducing it. When therapists feel that the pressure of managed care is further complicating their work with difficult patients, additional anxiety arises, thereby intensifying their own defenses and hampering treatment. Two common defenses I have observed therapists utilizing in the context of managed care are splitting and projection. Their feelings toward the patient are split, with all negative feelings projected onto the reviewer (Gabbard et al., 1991). This is destructive to the treatment, since therapists need the full range of their countertransferential feelings to understand and treat their patients adequately (Racker, 1968).

It is not only the therapist's countertransference that is profoundly affected by managed care's utilization review process—the patient's transference to the therapist is also affected. For example, many people come to therapy deeply mistrustful of the therapist and skeptical about his or her intentions and/or competence. Just the mere fact that the therapy has to be "managed" and "reviewed" compounds and reinforces these suspicions and transferential fears. And any doubts expressed by managed care about the validity or efficacy of the therapy is perceived as further confirmation of these mistrustful fantasies (Gabbard et al., 1991).

Since many patients utilize splitting as their principal mechanism of defense, cure is often based upon their integration of this split in the transference between "good" and "bad" aspects of the therapist. When a case reviewer interferes with the therapy, this healing process may also be interfered with, since the reviewer then becomes the target of the patient's bad internal object representations, thus promoting and intensifying the patient's preexisting propensity toward splitting. This deflects the splitting away from the transference, creating an obstacle to its systematic resolution (Gabbard et al., 1991).

As many psychoanalysts have observed (Kernberg, 1975; Searles, 1986; Spotnitz, 1984), preoedipally fixated patients are filled with rage, which often becomes displaced onto the therapist. Due to their need for vengeful aggression against their parents, they frequently enact self-defeating patterns that are transferred onto the therapist, resulting in an unconscious desire to defeat the therapist and destroy the treatment (Rosenthal, 1987). Pressuring them to improve, as managed care dictates, only conveys to them that they are bad and defective, which then intensifies their desire to sabotage the therapy in direct proportion to the therapist's demand for improvement (Gabbard et al., 1991).

CASE ILLUSTRATION

Because of the model espoused by managed care, psychodynamic psychotherapists working within this framework are pressured to alter their approach and abandon many psychoanalytic principles of treatment. The following is just such an example:

> John M., an overweight 13-year-old asthmatic patient, was referred to me by his managed care company due to his intense fears of the dark and an inability to sleep without his mother or to shower while she was not in the bathroom, fearing a stranger would break in and assault him. It was he who requested the therapy and the case was certified for ten sessions by his managed care company with their instructions that I should see other family members when necessary. Being slightly familiar with this company, I knew that if I could prove it was a medical necessity, at best the case would be recertified for an additional ten sessions.
>
> The patient's mother accompanied him to every session and seemed upset that he chose not to include her in his sessions. She was highly suspicious about what John told me about her and what I was revealing in my reports to the managed care company. On the one occasion I met with her alone, she revealed that she was born in Ireland, an only child like John, and had a very close symbiotic relationship with her mother, whom she continued to see on a daily basis. Her husband, although currently sober, had a history of alcoholism and was verbally "explosive." Although she was highly contemptuous of him and had her share of psychological problems (which she denied), she was uninterested in either individual or marital therapy.
>
> Immediately after my initial session with John, I started receiving numerous messages on my answering machine from his father that felt somewhat menacing, inquiring as to what John and Mrs. M. were telling me about him and requesting an appointment to tell me the "truth" about their situation. Although John knew of these calls, he did not want me to meet his father because he felt "embarrassed" and intruded upon. However, after a couple of months of persistent badgering and threats from Mr. M., and because of John's increased security in our relationship, he suggested that I meet with his father.
>
> As I suspected, Mr. M. was quite paranoid and blatantly psychotic. He was primarily concerned about what John and Mrs. M. had told me about him, and told me that Mrs. M. and John were

very close and disrespectful of him and often conspired against him. For the past three years he had been on psychotropic medication prescribed by a psychiatrist; he also wanted psychotherapy to help resolve his marital problems but felt that his psychiatrist was discouraging him from seeking therapy.

From the data I collected it was obvious that John was symbiotically attached to his mother, an attachment he felt ambivalent about, which is what originally brought him to my office. His father received the bad-object projection, while his mother was the idealized, nondifferentiated good object, from whom he could not separate, especially in their home, due to paranoid fears of his father as well as castration anxiety emanating from an oedipal sexualization of the earlier, preoedipal object-relations theme.

Feeling emasculated by these fears, John entered therapy with the goal of physically separating from his mother. Considering the severity of his and his parents' psychopathology, this was not a goal that could be realistically accomplished within our 20-session limit.

Achieving this goal was further complicated by the strong persecutory anxiety John experienced while in my office, partly based upon a negative experience the year before with a behavior therapist who immediately pressured him to separate from his mother. As a result, much of my attention was focused upon our therapeutic alliance and helping him feel safe and secure in my presence. Constantly keeping in mind that I was working within a short-term managed care model, my attention was also directed toward the therapeutic goal of helping John separate from his mother.

Feeling pressured to accomplish this goal before the expiration of our allotted 20 sessions, on our 17th session when John emphatically announced his desire to discontinue sleeping with his mother and to have her present at his next session to inform her of this, I hastily agreed, although I was keenly aware that I had not adequately resolved his and certainly not his mother's underlying resistances to such a separation. However, since I was influenced by the specter of managed care and was following the principles of "time-effective psychotherapy," I decided to risk such a meeting.

At that session, John informed his mother of his desire to discontinue sleeping with her and implored her not to respond to his pleas to the contrary. Although she cited numerous reasons why this could not be accomplished, she reluctantly agreed to try it that night. She also discussed her concern about her husband's "explosive" behavior, and I agreed to refer him to their managed care company for a reevaluation of his medication and for psychotherapy.

During the week following that session, I received a series of threatening phone calls from Mr. M., accusing me of telling his wife he was "crazy" and needed psychotherapy, followed by a phone call from Mrs. M., informing me that she was terminating John's therapy and that her attempt that night to help him discontinue sleeping with her failed miserably, since he cried and insisted that she sleep with him. She seemed angry, and I believe that through projective identification, Mrs. M. was expressing her rage toward me for abruptly interfering with her symbiotic relationship with John.

As I suspected, neither John nor his mother was ready to separate, and merely focusing on their manifest behavior rather than on their underlying character structures was of limited value. Based upon the progress the patient had already made, there is every reason to believe that if I had been able to proceed with this dyad at a slower and more cautious pace, with greater respect for my patients' underlying character resistances, these and other symptoms as well could have been alleviated. However, the pressures of managed care encumbered my usual approach to treatment, resulting in an unsatisfactory termination.

CONCLUSION

Psychodynamic psychotherapy is a comprehensive approach to the treatment of symptoms, since it focuses on the resolution of conflicts within the underlying character structure. This is in direct contrast to managed care, whose only focus is on the behavioral manifestations of these symptoms and their alleviation (Goodman et al., 1992). Managed care has lost sight of the fact that it takes considerable time for most patients to unlearn old behavioral patterns and learn new ones, since the preferred model of treatment is either short-term psychotherapy or medication for the alleviation of these symptoms.

Also disregarded by managed care is the relationship between patient and therapist, confidentiality in this relationship, and the establishment of a secure therapeutic contract, all of which psychodynamic psychotherapists consider essential for successful therapy. While managed care case reviewers can be sensitive and helpful to the therapist, these reviewers—often due to their demeanor and excessive concern with fiscal control—can also add to the therapist's difficulties in working with the patient. For these reasons many of the fundamental principles of psychodynamic psychotherapy are not only different from but also incompatible with those of managed care.

Psychodynamic psychotherapists are well aware that the insurance industry needs to establish a cost-effective system to cover the expenses of outpatient psychotherapy. Many believe that patients would be better served by a "cap" on annual reimbursements rather than by managed care (Graham, 1992; Shore, 1992). Since many psychotherapists utilize a sliding scale (Shore, 1992), an equitable fee based upon the patient's income and circumstances could then be negotiated, and a stable treatment frame could be established free of utilization reviews.

Although psychoanalytic psychotherapy is the oldest, best-studied, and most widely practiced form of psychotherapy (Kavanaugh et al., 1994), managed care disregards many of its most important concepts, which are indispensable for effective treatment. Although historically psychoanalysis has had numerous detractors, none has been as powerful or influential as big business. Since big business now exerts such pervasive control over mental health practice and practitioners, psychodynamic psychotherapy may be in danger of extinction.

ACKNOWLEDGMENTS

Parts of this chapter are based on the author's article "Managed care versus psychoanalytic psychotherapy: Conflicting ideologies," *Clinical Social Work Journal*, Summer 1994, pp. 37–148. The author would like to thank Andrea Labis, M.S.W., for her helpful suggestions and careful review of this chapter.

REFERENCES

Alperin, R., & Hollman, B. (1992). The social worker as psychoanalyst. *Clinical Social Work Journal, 20*, 89–98.

A.P.A. (1994). *Diagnostic and statistical manual of mental disorders* (4th ed.). Washington, DC: American Psychiatric Association.

Applebaum, S. A. (1977). *The anatomy of change*. New York: Plenum Press.

Bachrach, H. M., Weber, J., & Solomon, M. (1985). Factors associated with the outcome of psychoanalysis: Report of the Columbia Psychoanalytic Center Research Project (IV). *International Review of Psychoanalysis, 12*, 379–389.

Blanck, G., & Blanck, R. (1974). *Ego psychology: Theory and practice*. New York: Columbia University Press.

Bleger, J. (1967). Psycho-analysis of the psycho-analytic frame. *International Journal of Psycho-Analysis, 48*, 511–519.

Bozzuto, J. (1992). Psychoanalysis in the world of managed care. Presented at the American Academy of Psychoanalysis, December, 1992.

Budman, S. H., & Gurman, A. S. (1988). *Theory and practice of brief therapy*. New York: Guilford Press.

Caligor, L. (1981). Parallel and reciprocal processes in psychoanalytic supervision. *Contemporary Psychoanalysis, 17*, 1–27.

Cohen, C., & Sherwood, V. (1991). *Becoming a constant object in psychotherapy with the borderline patient*. New Jersey: Jason Aronson.

Davenloo, H. (1978). Evaluation criteria for selection of patients for short-term dynamic psychotherapy: A metapsychological approach. In H. Davenloo (Ed.), *Basic principles and techniques in short-term dynamic psychotherapy* (pp. 9–34). New York: Spectrum.

Di Bella, G. A. (1986). Money issues that complicate treatment. In D. Krueger (Ed.), *The last taboo: Money as symbol of reality in psychotherapy and psychoanalysis* (pp. 102–110). New York: Brunner/Mazel.

Edward, J. (1992, June 13). Report to the Executive Board of the New York State Society for Clinical Social Work. Presented at bi-monthly meeting in White Plains, New York.

Fiscalini, J. (1985). On supervisory parataxis and dialogue. *Contemporary Psychoanalysis, 21*, 591–608.

Gabbard, G., Tetsuro, T., Davison, J., Bauman-Bork, M., & Ensroth, K. (1991). A psychodynamic perspective on the clinical impact of insurance review. *American Journal of Psychiatry, 148*, 318–323.

Garfield, S. L. (1978). Research on client variables in psychotherapy. In S. L. Garfield & A. E. Bergin (Eds.), *Handbook of psychotherapy behavior change* (2nd ed., pp. 191–232). New York: Wiley.

Giovacchinni, P. (1979). *Treatment of primitive mental states*. New York: Jason Aronson.

Goldesohn, S. (1986). Transference, counter-transference, and other therapeutic issues in a health maintenance organization (HMO). In D. Krueger (Ed.), *The last taboo: Money as symbol of reality in psychotherapy and psychoanalysis* (pp. 158–168). New York: Brunner/Mazel.

Goodman, M., Brown, J., & Deitz, P. (1992). *Managing managed care: A mental health practitioner's survival guide*. Washington, DC: American Psychiatric Press.

Graham, S. (1992–1993). Managed care: The problem and solution. *The Psychotherapy Bulletin, 27*, 16–18.

Horner, A. (1991). *Psychoanalytic object relations therapy*. New York: Jason Aronson.

Josephs, L. (1992). *Character structure and the organization of the self*. New York: Columbia University Press.

Kavanaugh, P. B., Danulaoff, L. D., Erard, R. E., Hyman, M. & Pallas, J. L. (1994). Psychology: A profession and practice at risk. A position paper adopted by the Michigan Psychological Association. Unpublished.

Kernberg, O. (1975). *Borderline conditions and pathological narcissism*. New York: Jason Aronson.

Kernberg, O. (1976). *Object relations and clinical psychoanalysis*. New York: Jason Aronson.

Kernberg, O., Burstein, E., Coyne, L., Applebaum, A., Horwitz, L., & Voth, H. (1972). Psychotherapy and psychoanalysis: Final report of the Menninger Foundation Psychotherapy Research Project. *Bulletin of the Menninger Clinic, 36,* 1–275.

Kernberg, O., Selzer, M., Koenigsberg, H., Carr, A., & Applebaum, A. (1989). *Psychodynamic psychotherapy of borderline patients.* New York: Jason Aronson.

Kohut, H. (1984). *How does analysis cure?* Chicago: University of Chicago Press.

Langs, R. (1982). *Psychotherapy: A basic text.* New York: Jason Aronson.

Mann, J. (1973). *Time-limited psychotherapy.* Cambridge, MA: Harvard University Press.

Marmor, J. (1979). Short-term dynamic psychotherapy. *American Journal of Psychiatry, 136,* 149–155.

Marshall, R., & Marshall, S. (1988). *The transference-countertransference matrix: The emotional cognitive dialogue in psychotherapy, psychoanalysis, and supervision.* New York: Columbia University Press.

Masterson, J. (1976). *Psychotherapy of the borderline adult.* New York: Brunner/Mazel.

Meehan, B. (1994). From "comfort" to chaos: Mental health insurance coverage in the 1990s. *Psychoanalysis and Psychotherapy, 11,* 212–228.

Modell, A. (1976). "The holding environment" and the therapeutic action of psychoanalysis. *Journal of the American Psychoanalytic Association, 24,* 285–308.

Racker, H. (1968). *Transference and counter-transference.* New York: International Universities Press.

Reich, W. (1933). *Character analysis* (3rd ed.). New York: Pocket Books, 1976.

Rosenthal, L. (1987). *Resolving resistance in group psychotherapy.* New York: Jason Aronson.

Searles, H. (1986). *My work with borderline patients.* New York: Jason Aronson.

Sifneos, P. E. (1972). *Short-term psychotherapy and emotional-crisis.* Cambridge, MA: Harvard University Press.

Shore, K. (1992). Platform on managed care: Regarding outpatient mental health benefits. Unpublished paper.

Spotnitz, H. (1985). *Modern psychoanalysis of the schizophrenic patient* (2nd ed.). New York: Human Sciences Press.

Stern, S. (1993). Managed care, brief therapy, and therapeutic integrity. *Psychotherapy, 30,* 162–175.

Talman, M. (1990). *Single-session therapy.* San Francisco: Jossey-Bass.

Wallerstein, R. (1986). *Forty-two lives in treatment: A study of psychoanalysis and psychotherapy.* New York: Guilford Press.

Weber, J., Bachrach, H., & Solomon, M. (1985). Factors associated with the outcome of psychoanalysis. *Report of the Columbia Review of Psychoanalysis, 12,* 127–141.

Weinberger, J. (1994). The efficacy of psychoanalysis. *Adelphi Society for Psychoanalysis and Psychotherapy Newsletter, 8,* 9–13.

Winnicott, D. W. (1965). *The maturational processes and the facilitating environment.* New York: International Universities Press.

CHAPTER 11

The Impact of Managed Care on the Psychoanalytic Psychotherapeutic Process

Joyce Edward

Within the past ten years or so, powerful insurance and managed care companies have assumed increasing control of mental health services. Profit-making corporations and business managers are increasingly determining the nature and scope of mental health treatment. The expectations and requirements of industry have begun to take precedence over those of the patient.

As individual therapists attempt to adapt in this climate, they are being placed in the position of abandoning their respective codes of ethics and compromising the therapeutic work they do. The right of self-determination, which has constituted both a means and a goal of our helping efforts (Pearlman, 1971) is giving way in a system that depends upon compliance to function. Unseen, unknown individuals who may or may not be therapists now determine whether a person may have treatment in the first place. Once treatment is authorized, business-oriented individuals—sometimes clinicians, sometimes not, and rarely persons with psychoanalytic training—are increasingly determining whom the patient may see, what type of treatment he or she may have, how frequently the patient may be seen, and for how long.

In order to access their benefits, patients must waive their right to confidentiality. The most intimate details of their lives are now discussed on the phone with unknown persons who bear no responsibility for their welfare. The right to privacy is disappearing. Some companies demand to see notes of sessions and in some instances require that their reviewers be permitted to sit in on sessions. Vast amounts of highly personal information are accumulating in data banks all over the country without anyone really knowing who may access this information now or in the future. The two most basic components of an analytic therapeutic process, the patient's ability to speak freely and the therapist's capacity to listen freely, are being seriously compromised. From the patients' side, recognition that unknown others are privy to their thoughts and a constant awareness that reimbursement may end before a troubling issue can be worked through are among the features that are likely to limit free association. Issues related to managed care serve as an ongoing source of distraction, interfering with the expression of the patient's endogenously determined thoughts and thereby diminishing the opportunity to gain access to the workings of the patient's mind. These distractions also lend themselves to purposes of resistance. Since managed care matters must be addressed, it is more difficult to show their defensive use. From the therapists' side, the regulations, demands, control, and intrusions imposed upon them often lead to strong counterreactions that interfere with the achievement of an open-minded listening stance and optimum attunement. For both patient and therapist, the therapeutic situation has become less "safe."

In order to demonstrate the pervasive negative impact of managed care on the therapeutic process, I turn to two case vignettes.

CASE ILLUSTRATION—MRS. PHILLIPS

Mrs. Phillips, an unusually attractive, bright, always punctual woman, had been in treatment for 4 months for a severe depression at the time of the session to be considered. She arrived 10 minutes late for this particular hour, breathless and with eyes downcast. Clearly something was amiss. I had, prior to her arrival, begun to feel slightly uneasy. Had I failed to recall a change of appointment? Had she experienced some mishap? Might she not be coming at all? With this thought I began to review our last session. In that hour, for the first time, she had revealed that when she was a little girl, she and her father had frequently viewed pornographic films together while her mother was at work. They had kept this a secret, and this was the first time she had told anyone. Having shared this information with me, she immediately denied that the events had any importance. She then turned to a highly detailed discussion of some minor work-related incident. When she finally paused for a moment, I commented that I thought perhaps she was focusing so intently on her work because talking about the movies had indeed had an effect, a rather disquieting one. Seemingly ignoring my comments, Mrs. Phillips continued with her account of still another work-related event until the end of the session.

As I thought about her lateness prior to her arrival, I had begun to question my intervention in the previous session, wondering whether it would have been wiser to have waited for another opportunity to address the matter further. Was I beginning to rush too much, recognizing that time was limited with managed care patients like Mrs. Phillips? I thought of Fred Pine's well-taken point (Pine, 1985) that in some instances it is more helpful to "strike while the iron is cold" (p. 153) than when it is "hot." Under managed care arrangements, the iron unfortunately is sometimes removed before it cools.

Ordinarily I would expect during the session, if indeed Mrs. Phillips arrived, that through her associations and behavior she would enable us to gain some grasp of what was transpiring. I would undertake to provide her with as safe a situation in this hour as possible in order to maximize her freedom to communicate both verbally and nonverbally. This would involve maintaining those analytic attitudes of neutrality, anonymity, and abstinence which Roy Shafer has noted as essential for the creation of a "safe" therapeutic atmosphere (Shafer, 1983). Mrs. Phillips would be encouraged to tell in her own words and in her own time what was on her mind. While Mrs. Phillips might need to me to help her—through a question, an observation, or some acknowledgment that I was there with her—"go on" with her thoughts, she would have the chance to tell her own story with as little intrusion from me as possible. For my part I would seek to hear her story both affectively and cognitively. Together we would search for the meaning of what was said and heard.

In other words, Mrs. Phillips would ordinarily have been encouraged to associate freely and I would have sought to listen with what Freud referred to as "evenly suspended attention" (Freud, 1912, p. 11). By this I understand him to have meant that I would have avoided directing my notice to anything in particular. While bearing in mind what I already knew about Mrs. Phillips, what emerged in the last session, and the general analytic knowledge I possessed, I would nonetheless attempt to listen with an open-minded listening stance. Thus I would be prepared to hear the "new" and the "unexpected" (Freud, 1912).

However, this was not to be an ordinary session. Earlier that morning I had received a call from the utilization reviewer of Mrs. Phillips' managed care company, informing me that her twice-a-week treatment was to be reduced to one session starting the following week. The reviewer, a therapist of a different discipline and orientation, and from her own account of many less years' experience than myself, had determined that there was no "medical necessity" for twice-a-week treatment. The patient was working steadily, managing her household, and giving no indication of the suicidal thoughts that had initially brought her into treatment. Indeed, according to the reviewer, less frequent sessions would be therapeutically preferable in that they would reduce what she saw as the patient's growing "dependency" upon me. The reviewer averred that there were current studies showing that patients seen once a week fared better overall than those who were seen twice a week. I did not inquire about the details of these studies lest the reviewer feel I was challenging her. Above all, "providers" have learned to be "friendly." The reviewer then went on to propose that if Mrs. Phillips felt the need for additional support, she could join a self-help group for women who love too much. Impressed by a comment in one of my past reports that Mrs. Phillips appeared unusually needful of a man's acknowledgment, she felt that the patient might be seen as addicted to men. If such a group was not available, an alternative might be a group for families of alcoholics. Since Mrs. Phillips' grandfather was an alcoholic, the reviewer thought that she suffered from a genetic disposition to addiction. I reminded her that neither the patient nor her parents had drinking problems, but it was the reviewer's view that addicted persons share similar personality configurations and the treatment for one addiction is likely to be applicable to another. Also proffered were the names of several self-help books to suggest to the patient.

My efforts to persuade the reviewer of Mrs. Phillips' need for a continuation of the current time arrangement were unsuccessful. Among the points I stressed was her irrational fear of childbearing, which conflicted with her growing conscious desire to become a mother. She was obsessed with thoughts about dying during childbirth. I explained that this was a complex problem and that it would take time to understand and work through the issues surrounding it. It was important to do the work as soon as possible. Time was running out for this 36-year-old woman. The reviewer acknowledged that that was a problem but not one that would alter her decision. (May I say, that though this reviewer did see this as a problem, in the case of another patient with similar problems, the reviewer suggested that probably it was not a good idea for the patient to have a child anyway.) Mrs. Phillips' reviewer suggested that I propose some alternative ideas for the patient to think about when she began to ruminate about having a baby. Only if Mrs. Phillips' functioning worsened would the company be willing to reconsider. Meanwhile I was reminded that I had the right to appeal the decision. However, the reviewer quickly noted that a second reviewer might not agree that even once-a-week sessions were absolutely necessary. Thus, I realized, an appeal might lead to termination rather than an extension of treatment hours, making it unwise to take such a step. I explained to the reviewer that I realized she was making a decision consistent with her company's policies. In the final analysis I appreciated that the decision was theirs and I would take no further steps. She immediately responded that the company was not making the decision about treatment. It was up to the patient and the therapist to make treatment determinations. She was merely disapproving authorization for reimbursement. It was as if there were no connection between the reimbursement and the patient's ability to avail herself of treatment. I was reminded of George Orwell's "doublethink" (Orwell, 1974). You may recall Orwell defined that form of communication as consisting of knowing and not knowing, being conscious of complete truthfulness while telling carefully constructed lies, holding simultaneously two opinions that cancel each other out, knowing them to be contradictory and believing in both of them (p. 32). As our talk came to an end, I thanked the reviewer for the suggestions she had offered me. She, in turn, commented that she knew I was a psychoanalytically oriented provider and though the company respected psychoanalysis, she advised me that my perspective was not one regarded as consistent with the demands of managed care.

After the call I began to question myself, feeling that somehow I had failed to adequately support Mrs. Phillips's treatment. What could I have said differently that might have persuaded the reviewer to authorize further twice-a-week sessions? The only information that might have made a difference I was not at liberty to share. From the start I knew that Mrs. Phillips was still emotionally involved with a man with whom she had had an extra-marital affair several years earlier. Two years after what was to have been the end of this relationship, he was continuing to follow her about and to press her to leave her husband. On more than one occasion he had become violent, threatening to kill both of them if she did not join him. She had, in fact, first sought treatment following an incident in which he had struck her, seriously injuring her. It was this physically abusive relationship and her suicidal thoughts that had made me recommend the twice-a-week arrangement at the start. It seemed to me that Mrs. Phillips might unconsciously be arranging to be killed. At the patient's request, however, this information had been withheld from the company. She feared that in some way it might get back to her employer, and since the man she was involved with was a fellow employee, their jobs might be placed in jeopardy. Was Mrs. Phillips unduly concerned about the possible loss of confidentiality or was she being appropriately self-protective? Most of us who are experienced with managed care would think the latter. Patients' names, not their numbers, are regularly used in phone conversations, and one cannot assume that confidentiality can be protected now or in the future. I then began to wonder whether there was anything further I could have said about Mrs. Phillips' work performance that would demonstrate need. Failures in that area are taken seriously by companies. With some reviewers as long as an individual can arrive at work and perform their duties nothing else matters. Yet we all know that some highly competent workers can be severely handicapped in other significant areas of their lives. It is not, for example, unknown to hear of individuals who have done serious harm to themselves or others described by their employers and co-workers as having been exemplary employees.

Finally I put these thoughts aside and began to consider how I might best deal with the decision. I was convinced of the importance of continuing the twice-a-week sessions and began to wonder how this might be arranged. Did the reviewer's comment, though, that another reviewer might not see the need for even one session a week suggest that the treatment might be terminated in the very near future? If so, should I be more cautious about addressing issues that required more time to deal with? Yet if we avoid issues, how effective can treatment be? Even before Mrs. Phillips had told me about the movies, I had begun to wonder about possible sexual abuse in her background. She had repeatedly though briefly spoken of how disgusting she found it to be near her father, how inappropriate were the passionate kisses he gave to all women, including her grandmother.

Fortunately I was prepared and able to make whatever adjustments might be necessary to enable Mrs. Phillips to have what I regarded as necessary time to work. How much more, though, would I need to reduce the fee in order to enable her to continue? She had often stressed how important the insurance reimbursement was. Indeed when she signed the waiver of confidentiality, she had expressed some concern as to what it might mean in the future, but she felt it was worth foregoing some privacy in order to gain the reimbursement. In thinking about a fee reduction, I thought of those patients whose fees I had already reduced. How many reduced fees would I be able to manage? More, of course, than my younger colleagues, who have families to care for, children to send to college, and in many instances further training and their own treatment to pay for.

Regardless of what determination I might eventually make about the matter, how, I wondered, should I best raise it today? How could I provide Mrs. Phillips with an opportunity to express her thoughts about the decision and to identify the meaning it would have for her? Eventually I concluded that there was no adequate therapeutic way to deal with the matter. I would follow my usual course of raising matters such as vacation time and so on at the beginning of the session so that she would have a chance to respond. My concerns about the managed care situation occurred prior to my wondering about Mrs. Phillips lateness and ultimately overshadowed my responses to that action. Whether I could have drawn on my thoughts and reactions and her associations and behavior usefully in this session, I of course don't know, but the business of managed care took precedence.

One can look at my ruminations over the fee as an effort, in part, to gain some control over what I could control as well as to defend against my rage. I was certainly aware that the telephone call had left me anxious, depressed, and angry. I felt demeaned, powerless, and doubtful of my own competency. I was aware of a sense of having failed the patient and of some barely perceived fear with regard to her response. I already felt like the mother of the past who I knew had been unable to protect the patient and her brother from an alcoholic father and who had incurred the patient's wrath.

My self-confidence was also diminished by the presence of an unknown, unseen overseer with the power to make the most fun-

damental decisions about the treatment. I believe this arrangement tends to undermine one's self-confidence at best, albeit to
varying degrees, depending upon the therapist. It is essential that
we monitor ourselves and our own work carefully. Technical errors associated with both countertransference and lack of skill are
ubiquitous. Ongoing self-supervision and continued education as
well as consultation with peers or more experienced workers are
obligatory at particular times. However, it is another matter when
credentialed professionals are involuntarily forced into a position
of being "supervised" by someone who is likely to be less adequately trained and experienced than themselves and, in the case
of psychoanalytically oriented therapists, who are apt to devalue
that particular form of treatment. Despite my many years of training and experience, I was forced to confront the fact that I was
no longer appropriately in charge of my clinical practice. I was
also somewhat anxious because of the review itself. Had I been
too assertive in advocating for the patient? Therapists who have
acted similarly have been dropped from panels.

When Mrs. Phillips finally arrived for the session I am about to
describe I was obviously burdened by what had transpired, more
preoccupied with my own reactions and less open to hers. I began the session by noting that she appeared a little unsettled and
that I suspected from her lateness, which was so unusual, that
she had some significant matters on her mind. However, I did,
unfortunately have a matter to bring up that we would have to
deal with in this session and I thought it best to raise it at the
start. Mrs. Phillips, in a somewhat irritated tone, replied that she
had overslept. If she seemed unsettled it was because she had
rushed to get to her appointment. What was the matter I had
in mind? In what I realized even as I was talking was an apolo-
getic, overly lengthy fashion, I shared what had occurred. My disagreement and displeasure with the decision were evident. After
I completed the explanation, Mrs. Phillips showed no particular
feeling, though I sensed that there was a certain amount of relief in being able to turn away from her own thoughts to the issue at hand. The questions, decisions, and reports that must be
brought up from time to time relative to managed care of necessity divert both patient and therapist from their inner determined thoughts, thus offering both partners an easily available
vehicle for resistance. This is a particularly difficult resistance to
deal with, for reality dictates that we must, as in this situation, address the managed care issues if treatment is to be reimbursed.

After some discussion, Mrs. Phillips decided that she would, for the next 2 months draw on a special savings account to pay for the second session. This would give us time and hopefully she would be further along at that point and perhaps would not need the additional hour. She did not want or need a reduced fee. She noted that she might have stressed her dependence on the insurance, but this was because she did not want her husband to pay for any part of her treatment. She had hurt him enough by having the affair and then revealing it to him. It was wrong to take anything more from him.

About 3 weeks after the incident with the managed care company, Mrs. Phillips advised me that she was feeling better and that she would like to end the treatment. She was experiencing a greater degree of closeness with her husband. They were planning to take their first trip together in 6 years and she had decided to change jobs so that she could avoid seeing her former lover. She felt that in time, as she and her husband grew closer, she would feel more comfortable about becoming pregnant. While certain aspects of Mrs. Phillips' decision can be seen as potentially positive, I regarded her leaving as an effort to deal with her difficulties through avoidance rather than resolution. I also felt that this was a transference acting out. Just as she wanted to distance herself from her unprotecting, weak mother, who could not offer her significant help, I felt she wanted to distance herself from me. Yet I was unable to help her understand what might unconsciously be contributing to her wish to end the treatment and concentrated my efforts in the last sessions on ending in a way that might leave her free to return.

As I look back on my work with Mrs. Phillips, I regard it as an unsuccessful treatment and I regret that I was not able to help her more. Yet when I heard that the company that managed her benefits was planning to terminate a substantial number of clinicians from their list, I had the thought that because of my brief treatment of Mrs. Phillips, I might be seen as someone who did short-term work. Thus was the system shaping me.

MRS. PHILLIPS AND THE IMPACT OF MANAGED CARE

Although personal countertransference and therapeutic errors resulting from insufficient knowledge and/or inadequate skills are very likely to have contributed adversely to the treatment, there is no doubt in my mind that the arrangements of managed care greatly compromised the work. First, the treatment conditions tended to replicate some of the circumstances that had contributed to Mrs. Phillips' difficulties in the first place. For example, the need to withhold certain information from the company in order to protect Mrs. Phillips left her in a position not too dissimilar from the one she had been in as a child when she and father kept a secret from mother. At the same time I was unable to safeguard her treatment, just as her mother had been unable to protect her. Then there was the coincidence of the session reduction following the patient's sharing of critical information about the pornographic movies. One could imagine this to have been experienced as a warning—look what happens when you go against your father's wishes! Whether this was actually so I don't know, of course. However, Mrs. Phillips terminated treatment very soon after this incident.

The fact that I had temporarily abandoned my analytic attitude was itself, I believe, threatening. I was neither neutral, anonymous, nor abstinent in the session reported. When not defensively maintained, these attitudes promote safety within the therapeutic situation (Schafer, 1983) helping to assure that neither the client's nor our own wishes or fantasies will be acted upon in the treatment—that we will not impose our own values, judgment, or desires on clients and that we will not use them for our own psychic purposes.

In retrospect I can see more clearly how I was using the patient in that session for my own needs. When, for example, I supported Mrs. Phillips' decision to contact her benefits manager to question the rejection of the twice-a-week session, I consciously thought I was supporting her self-assertiveness. However, unconsciously, I was encouraging her to "help me." This unfortunately is likely to have been experienced by her as a repetition of her mother's dependence upon her to serve as her caretaker. To the extent that she was aware of my anger, I also lent myself to being experienced as she once experienced her uncontrolled, inappropriately behaving father.

We all recognize that departures from the analytic attitude do happen. Sometimes they are the outcome of personal countertransferences, the awareness of which leads us to self examination or to seek consultation with another professional. Other of our responses can be understood as having been at least in part induced by the patient and as such may be used diagnostically (Casement, 1985) and turned to the patient's therapeutic advantage.

I suggest that now we are confronted with an additional set of reactions that are sometimes evoked by specific requirements of managed care as well as the adverse climate it creates. These are no less of a problem than are our personal countertransferences. Indeed many times they combine with our personal unconscious issues, leading to serious resistances on our part. In the case of Mrs. Phillips, my personal reactions to the managed care arrangement blinded me to very important matters. Only when out of the fray did I begin to see more clearly some of the points I have raised here.

Since this experience, which occurred early in my association with managed care, I have consciously striven to recognize and deal more effectively with my own responses. This is no easy task. At best it is difficult to distinguish those reactions that are the result of personal transference, those that constitute "diagnostic responses," and those reactions that result from the frustrations that therapists experience in today's unfavorable therapeutic atmosphere. Any one of our responses, of course, is likely to reflect a mixture of all three. As a result an unusual degree of self monitoring is called for to identify what is happening inside us and to continue to maintain our therapeutic attitudes. While continuous self-observation is always essential, an overpreoccupation with ourselves is likely to be detrimental to the work, interfering with our capacity to remain adequately attuned to the patient. The increased degree of self-control necessary to prevent us from acting out our frustrations may well inhibit our appropriate spontaneity and ease in sessions, leading to a certain stilted atmosphere in the treatment room.

CASE ILLUSTRATION—MRS. RICE

I turn now to another patient, Mrs. Rice, in an effort to demonstrate that even when managed care experiences are more benign, the system nonetheless impedes process and compromises treatment.

Mrs. Rice, a 39-year-old, married, childless businesswoman had been in treatment for a little more than a year at the time of the work reported. When she began treatment her benefits were not managed, and we were free to develop a treatment plan on the basis of what she perceived as her needs and what I considered to be clinically appropriate. It was clear from the original consultation sessions that Mrs. Rice was not a candidate for short-term crisis intervention. Chronically depressed since adolescence, incapable of engaging in sex with a husband she seemed well related to emotionally, too fearful she would be injured during pregnancy or childbirth to bear a child, unable to express her full capacities in work, frequently sabotaging her success, incapable of forming intimate social relationships, wishing to die in order to be relieved of her dysphoria, both Mrs. Rice and I recognized her need for intensive psychotherapy. Indeed, psychoanalysis would, in my opinion, have been the treatment of choice. This modality not being feasible for a variety of reasons, we began with two psychotherapy sessions a week. Mrs. Rice viewed this arrangement as allowing her the freedom to say what was on her mind, secure that she would have a chance to continue in a second session and thus deal more promptly with the feelings that her thoughts engendered. She also regarded this frequency of treatment as affording her the opportunity to attend to the work sooner rather than later.

After about 6 months, a company took over the management of Mrs. Rice's benefits. Her first review was conducted by a psychoanalyst who agreed with the original treatment plan. Several months later, another reviewer eliminated the second weekly session.

The session I share follows Mrs. Rice's week and a half absence from treatment due to an out-of-town business assignment. Before she left, we were dealing with the repercussions of what she regarded as a significant change in the way she was approaching this assignment. Unlike in the past, Mrs. Rice was well prepared. Her speech was written. Her travel plans and her clothing were arranged ahead of time. She was consciously pleased. Yet prior to her departure her thoughts had turned to the danger of a plane crash. Her newfound achievements seemed to her to portend disaster.

The week that Mrs. Rice returned, her outpatient treatment report was due. I had failed to realize this earlier and so had not prepared her ahead of time. It is my practice to involve each of my patients in formulating these reports, believing that they should have a chance to determine whether what is being said is something they feel comfortable about having in their records. Today, therefore, I advised her that we would need to complete the form either in this session or in our second session of the week. Mrs. Rice chose to work on the report during this hour. If resistance led to her selecting this session, resistance to spending therapy time doing the form as well as certain concerns about this particular report probably led me to wish to delay doing it. I was aware of being concerned about whether further authorization would be granted. Mrs. Rice was making progress but she still had a way to go. The managed care company had merged with another company, as is so often the case. The newly formed organization was assuming a more restrictive stance. Would her inability to function sexually and her fear of success in her work and her continued dysphoria, albeit lessened, constitute sufficient reasons for this company's continuance of authorization? During the last review, the reviewer had insisted that the patient and her husband seek sex therapy. However, when I informed him of the unfavorable experience the couple had had previously and their unwillingness to pursue this course again, the reviewer withdrew the recommendation. He had also proposed that I ask the patient to consult with a psychiatrist in order to seek medication. When he was reminded that a previously consulted psychiatrist had advised against medication, he suggested that we delay this consultation. Efforts to coerce patients into medication are reported throughout the country and I was concerned that another reviewer might now require that the patient obtain another psychiatric consult. I was also concerned that the slowness of this treatment, by the company's standards, might lead the reviewer to question our continuing. I have been advised, after working with a very troubled patient for a year of once-a-week sessions, that if I had not helped him in that time, I probably never would. Either the patient should seek alternative treatments or "give up."

I was further distressed with the new form that had recently been adopted by the company. It provided even less opportunity to convey the uniqueness of each person than the previous one. One had the choice of describing a patient, for example, as disheveled, bizarre, inappropriately groomed, or well groomed. None of these categories accurately described Mrs. Rice. While she was carelessly, somewhat sloppily dressed some days, there were other days when she was neatly and more attractively groomed. Her appearance varies, depending sometimes upon her view of herself. Sometimes her less attractive grooming serves as a defense against her wish to be attractive, which she can experience as dangerous, exciting, or wrong, depending upon what issues are foremost at the time. On still other occasions Mrs. Rice feels that it is safer to dress poorly in order to avoid the envy of others. She fears that those who envy her will want to acqure what she has, just as she has wished to appropriate what others have. How can I indicate this? And should I? The new form has, I suspect, been developed to save the reviewer's time, among other things. Will I annoy the reviewer by offering more detail? These and other concerns preoccupy me. My focus keeps shifting from Mrs. Rice to the unseen reviewer. I am aware that I am at some distance from Mrs. Rice and less tuned in. I work against this but I nonetheless am listening more in terms of the report that in relation to her needs. I begin to feel somewhat tense and am in touch with the resentment that this arrangement is stirring up.

Mrs. Rice too must focus on the task at hand. She is eager to insure the continuation of her benefits. While she probably could afford with some sacrifice to pay for two sessions, she has paid for her insurance and feels, I believe correctly, that she is entitled to the "unlimited" benefits that were outlined in the company's original prospectus.

Mrs. Rice's first contribution to this report occurs in response to a question having to do with her self-perception. She points out in a rather removed way that she still feels at times invisible, and this makes her feel alone. Were this a regular session, we would pursue what she means by this, but it is not and I leave it at that, realizing with discomfort, that I welcome her comment for I can draw on it to show her distress. In retrospect I believe Mrs. Rice was actually conveying how she was feeling at the moment alone, invisible to me as I focused on the evaluation. At the same time I don't believe she is unmindful that what she has said is of some importance to the report.

Mrs. Rice becomes more involved when we come to a question that asks what has been discovered about the patient's history that is new. She notes that while nothing new has been discovered, the way she views the past has been modified significantly. She has in particular realized how much she needed to distort her impressions of her parents and in so doing unduly focused on their negative attributes. As she has been able to recall some of the more positive characteristics, for example, of her father, she is able to feel more for him and to be kinder to this now elderly, infirm man. As a result she feels better about herself. After saying this she immediately turns to her continued difficulty with intercourse. As other fears have diminished, her anxiety about sex and her depression over being unable to give and gain pleasure have increased. I note to myself that she has spoken about her father and then of her problems with intercourse. Contiguous ideas are often connected (Arlow, 1979). However, we are working on the form, not following her thoughts therapeutically. I do not bring this into our work today. I am also cognizant that having pointed to a gain, Mrs. Rice may be feeling it necessary to remind me that she still has a serious problem. Both patient and therapist are aware that there must be evidence of sufficient progress to suggest that the therapy is effective while at the same time their functioning must be sufficiently inadequate as to indicate "medical necessity."

After 20 minutes of this 45-minute session, the form is roughly completed. Mrs. Rice knows what will be included; she says she is comfortable with it, and I advise her that if she has any second thoughts, we can alter it in the next session. As if this were the start of the session, we now both settle back in our chairs. There are a few moments of silence and then Mrs. Rice turns to a rather detailed consideration of a social gathering she had attended the previous evening. She was pleased with her own participation. She had reached out more than in the past. I try to regain my empathic stance and follow her thoughts carefully, but somehow she appears disengaged and uninvolved in what she is saying. I wonder why she says nothing about the trip, about which there was much to say earlier. I did not ask, however, feeling that it was important that at least in our final minutes she be left free to proceed without interruption. She continued to speak of the party until the hour was over. As she went out the door, Mrs. Rice said that she could understand my concerns about managed care. She knew from her own experience what it is like to have people make your work more difficult.

In this session it is clear that the requirements of managed care took precedence over the patient's needs. She was deprived of the opportunity to begin with what was on her mind. For purposes of a persuasive report, my own empathic resonance with her was blunted by both countertransference and counterresponses as well as by the need to scan what was being said in order to complete the report. Ordinarily I am capable of tuning in to metaphorical language, but it was not until Mrs. Rice had left the session that I recognized that her statement about feeling invisible and alone was a communication about what was transpiring in the session with me.

In the next hour Mrs. Rice began describing another incident from work. I then noted that she had left the last hour commenting on her understanding of the difficulties she perceived me to be having with my work as a result of managed care. She said she knew I hated this new arrangement. I am different when managed care matters come up. I let my feelings show. Seeing me like that makes her uncomfortable. I appear weak and under the domination of the company. Actually, she is ashamed to say it, but she enjoys seeing me in that position. I have to endure what she has had to endure all her life, feeling humiliated and demeaned. She felt good to see me having an experience like hers, for she thought it would help me understand her better. She recognized, though, that she also drew satisfaction from being instrumental in placing me in a weaker position, as others had done with her. However, she also needed me to be strong and capable, and she felt insecure to realize how little control I had over certain matters. She came back to my being angry and said that she feels as if I wanted her to be angry too. After a silence of a few moments, she noted with obvious discomfort that she experienced me as inviting a kind of closeness between us that was disquieting. It felt sexual, as if I were trying to seduce her. In time it became clear that the experience had in fact evoked memories, feelings, and fantasies associated with Mrs. Rice's mother, who up until her 14th year used to come in to Mrs. Rice's bed during the night after having fought with her father. This closeness with her mother was both desired and feared. In retrospect, her parting words could be understood as a way of telling me that I was making it harder for her.

My weakness and powerlessness also evoked other images of her mother. A chronically depressed woman who suffered a painful physical handicap, she was perceived as weak and powerless. Mrs. Rice on one hand derived satisfaction from experiencing herself as stronger, smarter, and more capable than her mother. On the other hand she never felt safe or protected with her. Instead, she felt it was her responsibility to protect her mother. Before managed care, Mrs. Rice had perceived me at times as more powerful, more confident, and more able than she and at other times as less strong, confident, and able in accordance with her needs and fantasies at any given moment. However, in general, up until the managed care company took charge, I believe she had a baseline view of me as sufficiently capable and as appropriately in charge of her treatment. Thus it was possible to help her more clearly see how at times her own unconscious fantasies caused her to misperceive me and misrespond to me. After seeing my fees lowered, my judgment questioned, and my professional recommendations overridden, it was more difficult to identify the transference distortions. In addition the change in my status during the treatment was itself threatening to her overall sense of safety. Who we are and what we do are important. Patients need their therapists to be reasonably strong, relatively contented persons. Our professional confidence and our sense of appropriate authority help to promote trust and contribute to our ability to provide a favorable holding environment (Modell, 1974). Just as a child draws on the strength of his or her parents, so do many of our patients on ours. Kohut (1971) in particular has helped us to see the importance of our patients being able, when necessary, to experience us as strong and powerful. How, if we are powerless, are we to lend ourselves adequately to their idealizing needs? If we are powerless, how can we help to empower them?

CONCLUDING COMMENTS

Therapists are not the only ones finding managed care incompatible with psychoanalytic psychotherapy. By now it is clear to most clinicians that psychoanalytic forms of treatment and analytically oriented therapists are frowned on by most managed care companies. If admitted to panels such therapists appear to receive few if any referrals from companies. Indeed many therapists with whom I am personally familiar, no longer include their psychoanalytic training and experience in their vitae, believing that it will prejudice companies against them.

As we can see, even if companies allow for psychoanalytically oriented treatments, their demands and arrangements interfere with the unfolding of a favorable psychoanalytically oriented treatment process.

If companies do favor psychoanalytically oriented psychotherapy, their demands and arrangements interfere with the unfolding of a favorable analytic process. As long as reports of personal matters are required and patients are unable to feel secure in terms of the constancy of treatment arrangements, they will find it more difficult to associate freely. As long as therapists find themselves prevented from fully utilizing their hard-won expertise and no longer able to make appropriate clinical determinations about the treatment, they will find it difficult to retain the degree of therapeutic composure that is requisite if they are to remain optimally attuned to their patients and to turn to therapeutic advantage what their patients say and do.

How are we to deal with this situation? Many therapists have had patients whose case became managed only after treatment was well under way. Rather than abandoning their patients, they have followed them into the system when permitted to do so. Some therapists have joined the system because they do not want to discriminate against those who are dependent upon insurance. Others have felt that by joining the system they may have a chance to alter it. Still others know of no other way to support themselves and their families and feel they have no choice but to make whatever compromises are necessary simply to survive. On the other hand many of our most experienced clinicians are beginning to leave the field.

We must face the fact that psychoanalysis and psychoanalytic psychotherapy are in crisis. We who know the value of these therapies will have to do more than we have done so far if we wish to preserve the best of our clinical expertise. It is not the first time that the demands of the marketplace have conflicted with the needs of people. Indeed, more than a hundred years ago at a National Conference of Charities and Correction, one of the speakers noted that "The social problem with which the whole civilized world is now wrestling is how to reconcile economic and ethical law—the claims of business and of humanity, the decalogue and the multiplication table" (Pearlman, 1971).

We must begin to act if we do not wish to see contemporary analytic therapies "vaporized" (Orwell, 1974) and if we did not want to see a return to the therapeutic techniques of a century ago. When Mrs. Phillips' reviewer told me to advise her to think of something other than her concerns about childbearing, she was taking us back almost a hundred years to a time when therapists sought to effect change primarily by advice, persuasion, and coercion. Such techniques did not work well then and they are unlikely to do so now.

REFERENCES

Arlow, J. (1979). The genesis of interpretation. *Journal of the American Psychoanalytic Association, 27,* 193–206.

Casement, P. J. (1985). *Learning from the patient.* New York: Guilford Press.

Freud, S. (1912). Recommendation to physicians practicing psycho-analysis. In J. Strachey (Ed.). *The Standard Edition of the Complete Psychological Works of Sigmund Freud,* volume 12. (pp. 111–120). London: Hogarth Press.

Modell, A. H. (1976). The "holding environment" and the therapeutic action of analysis. *Journal of the American Psychoanalytic Association, 24,* 285–307.

Orwell, G. (1949). *1984.* New York: Harcourt Brace Jovanovich.

Perlman, H. H. (1971). *Perspectives of social casework.* Philadelphia: Temple University Press.

Pine, F. (1985). *Developmental Theory and Clinical Process.* New Haven, CT: Yale University Press.

Schafer, R. (1983). *The analytic attitude.* New York: Basic Books.

CHAPTER 12

Restructuring Managed Mental Health Care

William G. Herron

In psychotherapy, time provides opportunities to make treatment effective. These opportunities served as a core argument for promoting the idea that with psychotherapy, more is generally better—a conclusion that also has research support (Howard et al., 1986). The down side to the use of time was that psychotherapy costs increased with the number of sessions and that patient usage tended on the average to be short-term (Phillips, 1988). The usage data suggested that short-term therapy could be valuable, particularly if that was what many patients wanted. In addition, the cost of psychotherapy was reduced, so brief therapy would be attractive on this basis to consumers and funders. Thus, while many therapists saw patients' behavior as an underutilization of treatment and therefore an obstacle to effective outcomes, another group of therapists saw it as a chance to promote a more cost-effective treatment model. They interpreted patient usage as an index of consumer satisfaction with the quality of treatment that, in turn, provided justification for the widespread employment of brief psychotherapies.

They found support in the overall rising costs of mental health services, despite the fact that the rise was due primarily to inpatient treatment of alcohol and drug abuse (Broskowski, 1991). The practice of psychotherapy had become increasingly dependent on employer-provided health insurance. With the increase in health costs, employers were eager to make reductions. Proponents of short-term psychotherapy offered that possibility with quality assurance, and brief psychotherapies have gained dominance as the treatment most likely to get significant funding.

In addition, a vehicle for implementation was waiting in the Health

Maintenance Organization (HMO) act of 1973, which institutionalized managed care after its origination in the early 1900s (DeLeon et al., 1991). The original intention of the HMO movement was to provide affordable, accessible care (VandenBos, 1993); and in so doing it mandated minimums, such as 20 sessions per year of outpatient psychotherapy. The minimum quickly became a standard for treatment funding, and long-term or unlimited psychotherapy lost more and more possibilities of support. A variety of managed care entities appeared and are now in place to ensure that employer-funded psychotherapy remains brief. The norm has been set, and accommodation has been recommended to psychotherapists as the best survival mechanism (Cummings, 1988; Richardson & Austad, 1991). Of course, there are dissenters, including the integrated care plan suggested by the American Psychological Association (Welch, 1992), as well as plans that deemphasize inpatient care and emphasize outpatient care (Lowman, 1991). However, these are really more liberal managed-care plans that do not directly challenge the concept of limited outpatient treatment as an acceptable standard. Also, despite their retention of limits, they are not proving to be popular plans because they exceed the limits already accepted by funders. The result is that managed care keeps increasing its restrictiveness, so that time is literally running out, and with it the possibilities that are available through time spent in psychotherapy.

Although psychotherapy has always been managed in some fashion, once it began to be covered by insurance as a health service, the current management policies and practices became particularly odious to a very large number of practitioners (Alperin, 1994). However, for their beliefs to have an impact on funders, it is necessary to demonstrate that there are better alternatives. The desire for accountability on the part of funders is understandable and appropriate, so that suggestions made in this article regarding the restructuring of managed health care are made in the context of cost containment. The first step in proposing restructuring involves demonstrating the lack of validity in the current philosophy of managed care. This is followed by a discussion of the levels of mental health that are possible in society. The paper then concludes by offering ways to fund mental health care for these different levels.

MANAGEMENT PHILOSOPHY

In a series of papers that include reviews of the literature regarding the cost and value of outpatient psychotherapy (Herron & Adlerstein, 1994; Herron et al., 1994a; Herron et al., 1994b; Herron & Welt, 1992), the major assumptions of managed care are debunked. First of all, there is no cost crisis in outpatient psychotherapy, nor is it likely that there would be such a crisis even if managed care were not restrictive. The most potent argument against the cost crisis is usage data, which have always shown low rates. For example, in 1987, only 15% of the users had more than 20 sessions. While that accounted for 65% of total psychotherapy costs, it averaged only $789. It would be possible to reduce costs further by limiting those people to less than 20 sessions, but what would justify such a limit, given the relatively low cost of their treatment? Furthermore, only 3% of the people in the United States had outpatient psychotherapy in 1987, and the cost was only 8% of all outpatient care (Wiggins, 1994). These figures are in line with what was reported in the past when Shulman (1988) noted that psychotherapy was underutilized and DeLeon and VandenBos (1980) reported only 4% of health care costs were due to outpatient psychotherapy.

The cost crisis is nonexistent, and no evidence has appeared to challenge that finding. When it was suggested that unlimited outpatient psychotherapy could be provided for without any significant cost risk to insurance carriers (Herron, 1992), the dissenting response was that due to provider's greed, outpatient benefits can be misused if they are not limited (Lowman, 1992). Of course, such benefits can be abused, but nothing other than anecdotal evidence has been forthcoming to establish misuse. The relatively limited amount of outpatient psychotherapy that takes place suggests that provider greed is also quite limited. Outpatient psychotherapy is just an easy target for cost containment because such treatment does not primarily involve life-or-death issues. In addition, given the relatively few consumers, complaints are unlikely to have much impact on policy, particularly when people rarely choose policies for mental health benefits that they do not expect to use (Rubin, 1990).

However, cost reduction on this basis may be illusory because the review policies of managed care tend to involve frequent contacts and in turn a reviewing staff, so it becomes difficult to reduce overall expenses when the service being reviewed would not be particularly expensive if it went unreviewed. Also, the medical offset benefits of psychotherapy (Cummings, 1988) make curtailment debatable.

This raises the question of how valuable it can be to reduce services prior to the point of their maximum effectiveness. General guidelines for dosage effectiveness suggest that 75% of patients will show their greatest improvement after 26 sessions and 85% after 52 sessions, with anxiety and depression responding more rapidly than borderline psychosis (Howard et al., 1986). This contrasts with the 20 sessions generally suggested by managed care as a safe limit based on usage data of 10 sessions as a maximum for effectiveness, with 10 extra if needed.

This underestimation of effectiveness continues to be substantiated in recent studies. For example, Shapiro and coworkers (1994) compared the effectiveness for depression of cognitive-behavioral and psychodynamic-interpersonal psychotherapies at 8 and 16 sessions. Improvement criteria were seven self-report measures that included symptom severity and social adjustment as well as self-esteem. In regard to the time differential, 16-session treatment was more effective than 8-session treatment for severely depressed patients. This argues against the use of any set time limit even for a specific disorder, such as depression, because the severity of the problem affects the need for greater duration.

Kopta and associates (1994) investigated the durations required for different symptoms to remit to normal functioning. This approach incorporates the idea that improvement is clinically significant when someone recovers to the point that he or she is more like a normally functioning person than a dysfunctional person. Using such a criterion, it is possible to estimate probabilities of specific dosages of psychotherapy that will be needed to bring about normal functioning for people with different symptoms.

Symptoms were grouped into three categories, the first two including distress symptoms, classified as acute or chronic, and including anxiety, depression, somatization, compulsion, intense emotionality, phobic anxiety, obsession, and interpersonal sensitivity. The third category comprised characterological symptoms, including hostility, paranoid ideation, psychoticism, sleep disturbance, and overeating. These groupings were formed on the basis of response rates to treatment. In general, symptom improvement rates were congruent with the previous findings by Howard and colleagues (1986) of the greatest improvement in the beginning of treatment. However, the three symptom clusters represent three different recovery rates, with acute distress responding rapidly, chronic distress being intermediate, and characterological symptoms responding slowly, with about 40% of the patients failing to have symptomatic recovery after 52 sessions.

In an attempt to answer the general question of the effective duration of therapy, an evaluation was made of the response rates of symptoms that were most frequently represented in the sample and were in the distress categories, resulting in 18 symptoms. Nine of these were manifestations of depression, four of obsessive-compulsiveness, two of anxiety, two of interpersonal sensitivity and feeling guilty. The point at which 50% of patients with these symptoms had recovered was 11 sessions, but the point at which 75% of the patients had recovered was 58 sessions.

These findings reinforce the idea that brief therapy will provide relief for certain symptoms for about half of a treatment group; but to reach either the same symptoms in more people, or more symptoms, or more people, longer-term psychotherapy is needed. Although clearly even one session of psychotherapy can be effective, reduced psychotherapy does not appear to be cost-effective because of its clinical limitations.

Managed care for outpatient psychotherapy focuses on providing a relatively limited quality of care that adheres to a usage standard as opposed to care that is attuned to different effectiveness rates. These rates need to be addressed to ensure appropriate dosage models. Thus Kopta and coworkers (1994) note that their dosage estimates are higher than those of Howard and colleagues (1986) but that the difference lies in different treatment goals. The latter used general improvement, which can be established more quickly than a return to normal functioning, which was the goal in the research of Kopta and associates (1994). In essence, different levels of mental health can be attained by different amounts of psychotherapy. In that sense, more is indeed better, and meeting the criteron of "medically necessary" that is commonly used by utilization reviewers is doing the least for patients. The probable result is that considerable symptomatology is left untouched, and while acute problems may be alleviated, there is a high risk of symptom return because patients remain vulnerable. This ignoring of the preventive aspects of psychotherapy and the insistence on an immediate focus, both characteristic of managed mental health care, are not even really cost-effective.

Unfortunately, the illusion of adequacy of care tends to be dominant, using usage data as the evidence of validity. For example, a recent evaluation of managed care acknowledges the emphases on brief therapies, even where there are expanded mental health benefits and even though it is recognized that certain patients are not responsive to short-term approaches. The justification for the limitations are that they are in accord with a national average of eight sessions per year (Resnick, Bottinelli, Puder-York, Harris, & O'Keefe, 1994). That they may be true, but utilization rates and effectiveness rates are, as demonstrated, markedly different, and for management to be justified it should emphasize effectiveness.

Proponents of managed mental health care do mention that it has problems, but they tend to portray these as a necessary part of adapting to what is acceptable practice (Austad & Berman, 1991). However, the time limits are not so easily dismissed, as can be seen from the description of a seminar designed to train clinicians to be effective in a managed care setting (Donovan et al., 1994). Emphasis is given to experiencing a "crunch" in practice management because the system demands rapid turnover to be efficient. When this occurs, the therapists experience anger and helplessness, but these feelings are viewed as reactions that should be overcome, as though the system's operative mode were indeed necessary. The specifics of such operation are that most of the time is spent in evaluating many patients and then using very brief (one or two sessions) treatments for acute, specific problems. This is termed primary mental health care, indicating that more may be needed, but by implication that more therapy is secondary because this is good enough. Managed care systems are operating as though triage were needed, presumably for economic reasons, and at the same time as though such limited care were sufficient. Neither assumption is correct. There is not a cost crisis in regard to funding greater durations of outpatient psychotherapy (Bak et al., 1992), nor is the amount of psychotherapy being approved for funding likely to be sufficiently effective, particularly for any individual over time. These points need to be emphasized in determining how the provision of psychotherapy can best be managed. Management is essentially a policy issue and is best understood in the context of possible desired levels of mental health that can be attained with the use of psychotherapy. Thus the next section explores the variable structures of mental illness and mental health.

LEVELS OF MENTAL HEALTH

Successful management of mental health care requires that the mental health needs of society be assessed accurately and, in turn, that these needs then be met sufficiently through the appropriate distribution of services. Need assessment involves establishing desired mental health goals that are functions of the problems requiring solution as well as the methods most likely to produce solutions. The assessment can be conceptualized in terms of three levels of mental health: *necessity*, *potentiality*, and *improvement* (Herron et al., 1994a; Herron et al., 1994b). The level of necessity is the basic level of mental health at which individuals can carry out the tasks necessary to maintain their lives. When symptoms are present to the point that people do not have this ability, then they can be considered in need of psychotherapy to restore or maintain their functioning. These symptoms can vary in intensity and frequency, as well as from person to person, but their common feature is a debilitating impact on functioning. The treatment required is also at a basic level that involves targeted brief interventions which will produce rapid restoration or maintenance of functioning.

Managed mental health care generally aims at this level, considering it sufficient and thereby creating a treatment norm that also endorses a limited norm of mental health. While admissions are made that this will not be sufficient for everybody, the exceptions are made in terms of levels of pathology rather than health. Thus it is conceded that people with certain pathology, such as borderline and psychotic disorders, may need more treatment, but they are considered such a minority that they do not pose a serious threat to the policy of limited therapy as a norm.

This policy misses the mark in two ways. The first is that even in terms of symptoms, more treatment is needed than is approved by managed care to achieve maximum effectiveness. The second is that limited psychotherapy pays no attention to the other levels of mental health, namely prevention and potentiality. Brief therapy concedes the possibility of reappearance of symptoms and problems, which will be met with more brief therapy if the possibility become reality. Thus prevention is relatively ignored, being left to the hope that some therapy now will be sufficient for enough people to eliminate significant reappearances. This is a dubious possibility, so that maintenance of a standard of minimal mental health as a desired goal for the society appears primarily founded on immediate economic gain for funders. It is a policy that would be justified only if the economic situation were indeed a crisis in regard to the cost of psychotherapy, but that crisis is a myth. Furthermore, by paying so little attention to preventive treatment, current managed care practices may well result in future costs above those that would accrue if psychotherapy was not made so time-limited.

At this point the argument could be made that disagreeing with the emphasis on briefer, less expensive treatment as a goal is poor social and economic policy. However, the disagreement here is not with that goal but with what can be accomplished with the methods now in place. The search for efficient models of treatment always needs to be operative, but it remains necessary to take issue with a policy that reinforces the idea that the least that psychotherapy can do is also the best that it can do. Also, asserting that the quality of care is related to the duration of psychotherapy is a policy statement about the goals of psychotherapy which unfortunately has led to the casting of ethical stones. Those providers favoring long-term psychotherapy have been termed greedy because they apparently want to retain patients beyond the time that is needed, or they have been considered uninformed and inflexible because they fail to embrace brief therapies as adequate solutions. As the same time, short-term therapists have also been called greedy because they can appear merely to be doing what funders want in order to get their money, or uninformed because they debunk the benefits of long-term work and convince patients to accept solutions that can be of limited effectiveness. Of course personal issues are involved, but it is both prudent and useful to focus on what mental health policy is desired by the society and how can that best be put into practice. If the society favors the level of necessity, then the promotion of a short-term model will predominate. However, it is doubtful that at the moment managed care policies are based on society's complete understanding of mental health needs—as illustrated below in examining the levels of improvement and potentiality.

The level of improvement builds on the level of necessity. It is designed to improve functioning once that is restored or maintained. The presence of depression is an example. If a person becomes so depressed that he or she cannot perform a basic life function, such as work, then that person is at the level of necessity. Once the depression has been alleviated to the point that the person can work, he or she is at an intermediate level of improvement. The depression can be further alleviated so that the job performance increases in effectiveness and other aspects of life are also improved, even though these improvements are not necessary for a basic level of functioning in these areas. Interventions aimed at this level are also more likely to be preventive because they are improvements in functioning. This intermediate level of improvement is a concept that managed care may even be forced to embrace if, over time, level-of-necessity interventions for each individual become frequent. It is also a concept that, properly explained to funders and consumers, is likely to have sufficient appeal that it would become the norm. In fact, the failure of managed care entities to make intermediate care the norm, and instead to utilize minimal federal guidelines as limits for maximum coverage, makes them vulnerable to criticisms that they are favoring cost over quality. For some immediate cost increases, they could offer a better rationale than "Our limits are sufficient because usage data averages less than what we offer." They could also avoid criticism by stopping the frequent utilization reviews and the doling out of preapprovals in six- to eight-session increments. These are costly and create antagonisms between the reviewers and both providers and consumers. The APA has suggested no reviews before 50 sessions (Welch, 1992), and again usage data suggest that it is a relative few in the patient population who will even use that number. Unfortunately for their mental health, patients are settling for less and managed care encourages this, but both groups could regret it in the light of effectiveness studies.

Finally, there is the level of potentiality, which stresses the educative and growth possibilities of psychotherapy. This is an expanded level, building on but going beyond necessity and improvement. This level stresses the idea "Be the best you can be." It has broad social goals, the creation of a citizenry that favors peace over war, altruism over greed, enlightenment over ignorance—in essence, enabling people to achieve their potentials. It is not medically necessary in the basic or even improvement senses, but it has a long-range ambition of the betterment of lives. As such it is time-consuming and expensive and requires considerable effort from consumers with less obvious increments of change as well as plateaus. The goal is lofty: namely, ideal mental health for as many people as possible. But its lack of immediacy, greater length, and greater cost make it unlikely that it will get significant funding. Still, given the value of potentials being actualized, it bears consideration on an experimental basis.

The layers of mental health have been represented over time in a compromise formation model (Herron & Adlerstein, 1994). The highest layers represent successful defenses against the anxieties created by policies in place at the time. The highest layers would reflect successful defenses, classed as sublimation, in which the goals achieved are experienced as satisfactory enough to keep the existing policy relatively intact. Satisfaction would be considerably above average, maintained by meeting the needs of funders, consumers, and providers sufficiently so that there would be few complaints or abuses. Policy review would be ongoing as well, so that dissatisfactions that appeared could be addressed. Flexible adaptation mechanisms would be used to effect compromises and preserve an attainment to shifting societal needs.

Psychotherapy has never been at this level, although it did operate in the 1960s and 1970s with a greater degree of acceptance and satisfaction from consumers, providers, and funders than has been the case since then. A major concern of the downward drift was the failure of providers to either make a credible presentation of the value of their services in the form operative at that time or have different delivery systems available that would meet with sufficient acceptance.

The result was the inception of the predominance of the next layer of compromise, in which there were less successful defenses providing more limited partial adaptation. The defenses present at this stage are often stalling operations that keep in check disturbing feelings without making significant changes. Repression, rationalization, and displacement can all be used to try to ignore the problem, resulting in, for example, providers failing to recognize the implications of the increased dependency of consumers on using insurance payments for psychotherapy. Denial of the value of long-term psychotherapy by funders is a more serious defense, along with the projection of aggression to providers as justification for the need to cut funding for psychotherapy. These defenses are all signals of serious policy problems and become apparent in the lack of unity in attempting to find solutions. Instead, there were attempts to either keep what was in place or destroy it, which has resulted in psychotherapy policy operating at the third, or symptomatic level, in which compromise is exacted in a painful, disruptive fashion.

The symptomatic level, which prevails at the moment, is marked by defensive failure and the breakthrough of overt dissatisfactions that signals the need for change. If changes are not made at this time, then there will be more suffering and turmoil, with the policy ruling by force until there is significant adaptation to move the policy back at least to the second layer, with the hope of returning to the level of sublimation. This is not going to happen by insisting that managed care in its current form is either necessary or effective when applied to outpatient psychotherapy.

The concept of levels of mental health has also been approached in terms of phases of psychotherapy. Three phases of psychotherapy have been suggested—namely, remoralization, remediation, and rehabilitation—which differ in their goals, methods of intervention, and durations needed to be achieved (Howard et al., 1993). This is based on a model of psychopathology in which a person finds a lack of psychological resources to cope with a particular life situation. As a result, the person's life functioning suffers to the point of symptom formation that then persists and results in a sense of helplessness. The person then has the need to seek psychotherapy, which sequentially reverses the pathology sequence.

Thus, the psychotherapy phases begin with the goal of addressing powerlessness and the lack of hope in order to enhance a sense of subjective well-being. This stage of remoralization emphasizes the creation of hope and can often be brought about quickly through a variety of interventions, some as simple as a person making an initial appointment for therapy. People who stop at this phase and are satisfied apparently feel they have established sufficient personal well-being to put coping mechanisms in place and resolve the precipitating decrements in functioning that stimulated seeking psychotherapy. Of course, there are also people who stop at this phase because they remain demoralized and consider the interventions to have been of no value. Usage data suggest that this first phase is typical for patients, whether it is effective or not. It is congruent with the basic level of necessity described previously as well as fitting the brief therapy model.

The next phase builds on remoralization to seek remediation for symptoms and/or problems in living. Attention is paid to the facilitation of coping skills, which is possible through a variety of interventions. Although this phase is designed to build on the first phase, some patients may begin with the need for symptomatic relief before they reach the stage of demoralization. This second phase is of greater duration than the first, although its length tends to be variable depending on individual symptom patterns and reactions to interventions. It overlaps the levels of necessity and improvement previously described. Many patients stop therapy when this phase has been completed, particularly if the symptoms abate quickly and do not make a rapid return.

The third phase of rehabilitation builds on the first two and involves patients who seek to change problematic maladaptive patterns in their lives that illustrate the acute distress that may have motivated them to seek therapy. This phase then emphasizes changing their disturbing repetitive patterns to new ways of living life that are more adaptive and satisfying. This is a more lengthy process that has educative and preventive elements, overlapping the levels of prevention and potentiality discussed earlier. This type of treatment is rarely supported by managed care on the grounds that it is not medically necessary. However, given its preventative components, it could certainly be argued that it is indeed needed to ensure the durability of health. In essence, medical necessity is not exclusively an acutely focused concept, and it is erroneous to use it that way.

Some patients may enter psychotherapy in this phase if their concern is more of a holistic psychoeducational one than a response to acute problems, but the process is still focused on their mental health. Also, maintaining gains or preventing relapses may be part of this phase. Although some exceptions have been noted, the usual pattern is for patients to begin with the need for remoralization, and if therapy continues, for this to be followed by remediation and rehabilitation.

Howard and colleagues (1993) tested the accuracy of this model by measuring patients' functioning at intake, sessions 2 and 4, and session 17. The measures included subjective well-being to reflect phase one, symptomatic distress for phase two, and current life functioning for phase three. Six life areas measured were family functioning, interpersonal relationships, intimate relationships, work, health and grooming, and self-management.

Howard and associates (1993) found that at termination, 85% of the patients had improved their subjective well-being, with a significant amount of improvement occurring by session 2. For symptomatic distress, 74% of the patients had improved by termination, and the improvement rate decreased to 67% for current life functioning. Thus the achievement of goals takes longer as their scope increases, and less people are improved in the same time span when the goals are expanded. Causal analyses indicated the frequency of a sequence of improvements in well-being, reduction in symptoms, and improved life functioning. At the same time, improvement in subjective well-being was not sufficient for symptom reduction, nor was symptom alleviation sufficient for improvement in life functioning. Thus, there is no justification for asserting that the goals of brief therapy when achieved will generalize to other goals, such as the improvement of life functioning. On the contrary, the evidence suggests that although brief therapy can do its job, that job is a restricted one that fails to meet other levels of mental health that also could be described as medically necessary.

The model of levels of mental health appears as the most rational approach to developing funding policies for psychotherapy. The "one size fits all" or "fits enough" approaches that have characterized managed mental health care are lacking in quality of care when they are applied to the need for levels of mental health that go beyond basic necessity. Because these levels are of greater value than current funders and policy makers acknowledge in promoting their form of health care, it is essential to restructure managed care to make provisions for different goals than are currently being emphasized.

NEW DIRECTIONS

In general there is a desire among funders to regulate all forms of health care in order to provide the greatest possible cost control. This desire includes the regulation of outpatient psychotherapy even though its costs are minor compared to other health services. It has been possible to effect immediate cost reduction by reducing both the amount paid per session and the number of sessions of psychotherapy, but there is a limit to how much reduction is possible, particularly given an average use of eight sessions per year without managed care and utilization review. It is also clear that the temporal limitations being imposed are also qualitative limits, which deny access to other, better levels of mental health. As a result, a major target for restructuring is time limits.

How can this be accomplished without excessive cost? By beginning with the recognition that even unlimited outpatient psychotherapy benefits would not be particularly costly because not that many people would use such benefits. In addition, Haas and Cummings (1991) noted that such a policy would be clinically and ethically correct, although they considered it an economic risk. However, they stated, "Although this is not a widespread policy . . . it has proven viable when carefully implemented" (p. 47).

The cost uncertainty is always raised as an objection by opponents of the possibility (Lowman, 1992), as though it actually had been proven that costs would be excessive, but it has not. In fact, unlimited outpatient coverage has rarely even been attempted. Managed care is not a limitation of the previously limitless but rather further limitation of the limited, because mental health coverage always had limits and coverage was always more restricted than it was for other health conditions.

Is it possible that some patients and therapists might collude to unnecessarily prolong psychotherapy if cost were not an issue? Of course it is possible, but it is also unlikely, other than infrequently. The reasons are ethical and legal constraints in regard to quality of care—namely, that unnecessary treatment is not acceptable, and on a practical level, patients in the main are not interested in lengthy therapy. They actually and understandably prefer brief treatment. As all therapists know when they have been faced with what they see as premature termination, it is either difficult or impossible to deter such patients.

In contrast, it would be rather easy to convince many patients that they are fine after a short course of treatment because gains tend to be larger in the beginning and because it is what most patients would like to hear. However, it could be ethically risky if indeed they are being cut off to restrict costs; and if they ultimately get worse, it could be costly. So brief therapy has economic risks as well.

Unlimited outpatient psychotherapy benefits accompanied by careful monitoring of both usage and outcome ought at least to be given a substantial trial. If the minor economic risk in that approach seems too radical to funders at a time when immediate cost cutting is so popular, then at best they could open up the benefits to allow for maximum effectiveness to one year of outpatient psychotherapy before imposing limits, because there is clearly a clinical risk in the insistence on brief psychotherapies, and that clinical risk is potentially costly. Employers discovered the ultimate cost of immediate returns in regard to environmental disregard, so that lesson could be well applied in regard to outpatient mental health services. After all, it is not as though outpatient mental health benefits were ever particularly generous, but now the situation has degenerated. As that becomes more apparent, it adds to the idea that it would really be better for mental health benefits to be redesigned to provide for more outpatient psychotherapy than was available before managed care became so prevalent. Actually, the concept of benefit redesign to favor outpatient over inpatient care is gaining popularity (Lowman, 1994), but it is still linked with improving economic limits on the duration of outpatient psychotherapy, which unfortunately perpetuates a myth of unending therapy and unlimited cost.

Thus, the most basic proposal made here is that the management of mental health care consider the expansion of outpatient coverage to the point of an unlimited number of sessions as both the most economical and clinically effective way to operate. Such an approach would be monitored, with accountability expected, and, if proven to be ineffective, then adjustments would have to be made. In the process, monitoring needs to be observational, done only at appropriate intervals, and not coercive; furthermore, accountability needs to be congruent with agreed upon goals that reflect sought after levels of mental health. For example, Luborsky and coworkers (1993) indicate how psychological health-sickness (PHS) can be measured and its applicability to different psychotherapeutic orientations. In turn, different levels of PHS are reflective of different treatment goals, so that there are existing ways to monitor effectiveness that do not have to disregard certain clinical orientations and objectives. Therapists are not averse to offering treatment plans or establishing accountability provided that these are congruent with the level of mental health that is the goal. Of course, to achieve such congruence, it is necessary to have an acceptance of the goals by funders, consumers, and providers. At the moment, the goals are restricted to the basic level, so clearly that needs to be changed and then the restrictiveness and immediate gratification now in place would no longer be considered of value.

In addition to the insistence on brief psychotherapies, there are a number of other restrictive tactics used by managed care that clearly seem to be designed to curtail usage and thereby limit costs regardless of service quality. Utilization review (UR) is one example, where often a separate entity is created for periodic consultation by the providers in order to gain approval of the number of sessions to be covered. This is usually done at frequent intervals—for example, every four sessions—and has an adversarial quality about it in that the provider and the patient are expected to justify every continuance. In addition there may also be a plan administrator who disburses payment, adding more management. At a time when many companies are downsizing, it seems paradoxical that these same companies believe money will be saved through the creation of more layers of personnel to manage their health plans.

Another obstacle is the restriction of patients' choice of providers and the restriction of providers from plans. Although managed care often claims it is managed competition, the aim seems to be to restrict competition. Shore (1994) documents the restrictive practices of managed care and suggests alternatives that essentially provide for the freedom of choice that is particularly important in psychotherapy, where the fit between patient and therapist is generally considered a necessary component of effectiveness.

The restructuring of managed care ought to be put into operation as soon as possible, with its central theme being the reduction of management. Policies that provide extensive outpatient coverage should be encouraged, along with the choice of providers. Traditional copayments, varying from 20 to 50% are workable, as are lifetime caps, provided that fees are negotiated between patient and therapist. Whether short- or long-term therapies will be most popular could then be decided by consumers, not by outside parties who have the most to gain from one type of therapy. There is evidence that brief therapies are not sufficiently effective, but there is no evidence that freedom of choice in regard to length of outpatient psychotherapy or providers will result in excessive costs. The logical conclusion is that options ought to be made available so that the results can be evaluated prior to enshrining the need for managed outpatient psychotherapy in its current form. It is fascinating in a macabre fashion that at the moment the people most affected by managed care—consumers and providers—have had the least to do with either its origination or its implementation.

It is difficult to discuss the funding of any type of health care without considering the funding of all health care, because funding policies tend to be created as overviews that subsequently address specifics. Then, although the concern here is with outpatient psychotherapy, the funding for that usually comes from the general category of mental health benefits, which is one segment of all health benefits funded either by employer–employee contributions or government programs based on taxation (French & VandenBos, 1994). Keeping that big picture in mind, cost savings alternatives to managed care have been suggested, such as medical savings accounts, managed cooperation (Shore, 1994), and deductibles based on income (Herron & Welt, 1992). However, a different point is being made here, namely, that the type of managed care being applied currently to outpatient psychotherapy is an economic mistake. As a result it could be either deleted or severely curtailed and the money now spent on management would be saved.

Specifically, all insureds could be allowed up to 50 outpatient sessions per year with 80% coverage on fees up to $100 per session without creating a cost problem. The level of necessity will be covered for most people, and the level of improvement will at least have been initiated. Putting the approach into place makes it possible to see how many sessions are used. In addition, all insureds who are using psychotherapy could also indicate any need or desire to continue psychotherapy after 50 sessions, thus providing an indication of the demand for more extensive therapy. Psychotherapists are there to serve and in turn to make a living through that service. They have always worked with patients' economic situations and will continue to do so, but they cannot do the best for their patients when the best is mandated as the least. Effectiveness and time are related, not eternally, but for more than the current practice of managed care allows. Just as their advocates once warned providers of the dangers of ignoring the emphasis on brevity, the warning is now sounded as to the dangers of that very emphasis.

REFERENCES

Alperin, R. M. (1994). Managed care versus psychoanalytic psychotherapy: Conflicting ideologies. *Clinical Social Work Journal, 22,* 137–148.

Austad, C. S., & Berman, W. H. (Eds.). (1991). *Psychotherapy in managed health care: The optimal use of time and resources.* Washington, DC: American Psychological Association.

Bak, J. S., Weiner, R. H., & Jackson, L. J. (1992). Managed mental health care: Should independent private practitioners capitulate or mobilize? *The Independent Practitioner, 12,* 31–35, 75–80, 159–164.

Broskowski, A. (1991). Current mental health care environments: Why managed care is necessary. *Professional Psychology: Research and Practice, 22,* 6–14.

Cummings, N. A. (1988). Emergence of the mental health complex: Adaptive and maladaptive responses. *Professional Psychology: Research and Practice, 19,* 308–315.

DeLeon, P. H., & VandenBos, G. R. (1980). Psychotherapy reimbursement in federal programs: Political factors. In G. R. VandenBos (Ed.), *Psychotherapy: Practice, research, policy* (pp. 71–102). Beverly Hills, CA: Sage.

DeLeon, P. H., VandenBos, G. R., & Bulatao, E. Q. (1991). Managed mental health care: A history of the federal policy initiative. *Professional Psychology: Research and Practice, 22,* 15–25.

Donovan, J. M., Steinberg, S. M., & Sabin, J. E. (1994). Managed mental health care: An academic seminar. *Psychotherapy, 31,* 201–207.

Frank, R. G. & VandenBos, G. R. (1994). Health care reform: The 1993–1994 evaluation. *American Psychologist, 10,* 851–854.

Haas, L. J., & Cummings, N. A. (1991). Managed outpatient mental health plans: Clinical, ethical, and practical guidelines for participation. *Professional Psychology: Research and Practice, 22,* 45–51.

Herron, W. G. (1992). Managed mental health care redux. *Professional Psychology: Research and Practice, 23,* 163–164.

Herron, W. G., & Adlerstein, L. K. (1994). The dynamics of managed mental health care. *Psychological Reports, 75,* 723–741.

Herron, W. G., Eisenstadt, E. N., Javier, R. A., et al. (1994a). Session effects, comparability, and managed care in the psychotherapies. *Psychotherapy, 31,* 279–285.

Herron, W. G., Javier, R. A., Primavera, L. H., & Schultz, C. L. (1994b). The cost of psychotherapy. *Professional Psychology: Research and Practice, 25,* 106–116.

Herron, W. G., & Welt, S. R. (1992). *Money matters: The fee in psychotherapy and psychoanalysis.* New York: Guilford Press.

Howard, K. I., Kopta, S. M., Krause, M. S., & Orlinsky, D. E. (1986). The dose-effect relationship in psychotherapy. *American Psychologist, 41,* 159–164.

Howard, K. I., Lueger, R. J., Maling, M. S., & Martinovich, Z. (1993). A phase model of psychotherapy outcome: Causal mediation of change. *Journal of Consulting and Clinical Psychology, 61,* 678–685.

Kopta, S. M., Howard, K. I., Lowry, J. L., & Beutler, L. E. (1994). Patterns of symptomatic recovery in psychotherapy. *Journal of Consulting and Clinical Psychology, 62,* 1009–1016.

Lowman, R. L. (1991). Mental health care claims experience: Analysis of benefit redesign. *Professional Psychology: Research and Practice, 22,* 52–59.

Lowman, R. L. (1992). Managing mental health care wisely: More is not necessarily better. *Professional Psychology: Research and Practice, 23,* 164–166.

Lowman, R. L. (1994). Managed mental health care: Critical issues and next directions. In R. L. Lowman & R. J. Resnick (Eds.), *The mental health professional's guide to managed care* (pp. 169–180). Washington, DC: American Psychological Association.

Luborsky, L., Diguer, L., Luborsky, E. H., et al. (1993). Psychological health-sickness (PHS) as a predictor of outcomes in dynamic and other psychotherapies. *Journal of Consulting and Clinical Psychology, 61,* 542–548.

Phillips, E. L. (1988). Length of psychotherapy and outcome: Observations stimulated by Howard, Kopta, Krause, and Orlinsky. *American Psychologist, 43,* 669–670.

Resnick, R. J., Bottinelli, P. W., Puder-York, M., et al. (1994). Basic issues in managed health services. In R. L. Lowman & R. J. Resnick (Eds.), *The mental health professional's guide to managed care* (pp. 41–62). Washington, DC: American Psychological Association.

Richardson, L. M., & Austad, C. S. (1991). Realities of mental health practice in managed-care settings. *Professional Psychology: Research and Practice, 22,* 36–44.

Rubin, J. (1990). Economic barriers to implementing innovative mental health care in the United States. In I. M. Macke & R. A. Scott (Eds.), *Mental health care delivery: Innovation, impediments, and implementation* (pp. 220–232). New York: Cambridge University Press.

Shapiro, D. A., Barkham, M., Rees, A., et al. (1994). Effects of treatment duration and severity of depression on the effectiveness of cognitive-behavioral and psychodynamic-interpersonal psychotherapy. *Journal of Consulting and Clinical Psychology, 62,* 522–534.

Shore, K. (1994). Managed care and utilization review. *Psychologist Psychoanalyst, 14,* (4), 5–9.

Shulman, M. E. (1988). Cost containment in clinical psychology: Critique of Biodyne and the HMOs. *Professional Psychology: Research and Practice, 19,* 298–307.

VandenBos, G. R. (1993). U.S. mental health policy: Proactive evaluation in the midst of health care reform. *American Psychologist, 48,* 283–290.

Welch, B. (1992). The best care: Integrated, not managed. *The APA Monitor, 23,* 30.

Wiggins, J. C. (1994). How study supports psychotherapy but challenges psychologists. *Psychotherapy Bulletin, 29,* (3), 45–46.

Name Index

Subject Index